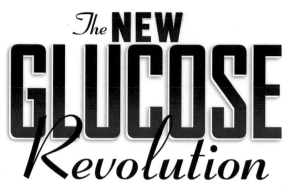

Low GI Vegetarian Cookbook

80 Delicious Vegetarian and Vegan Recipes Made Easy with the Glycemic Index

Dr. Jennie Brand-Miller • Kaye Foster-Powell
Kate Marsh • *with* Philippa Sandall

Marlowe & Company • New York

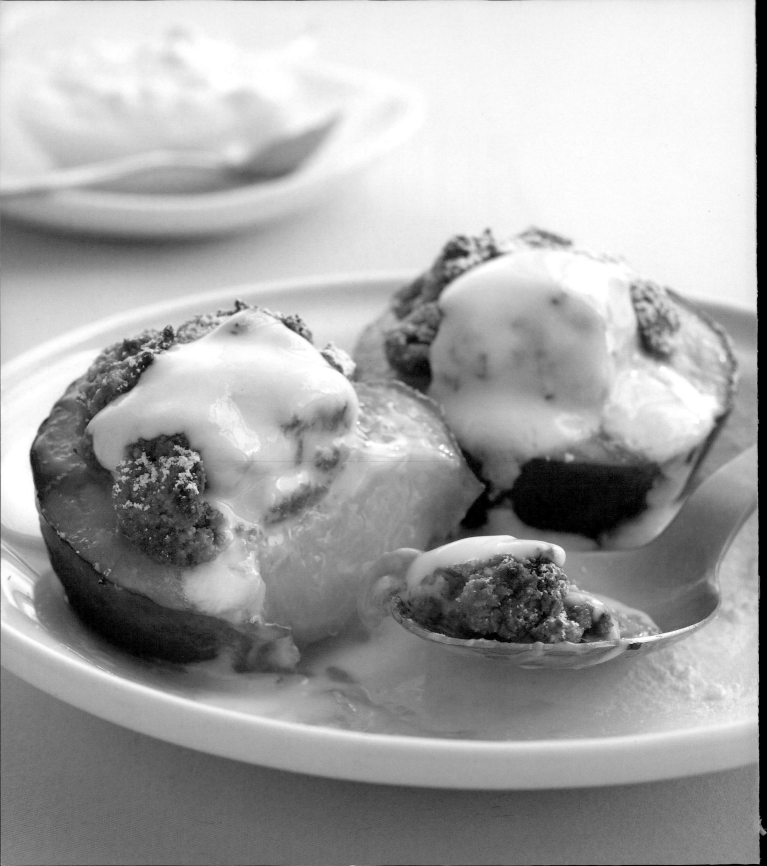

contents

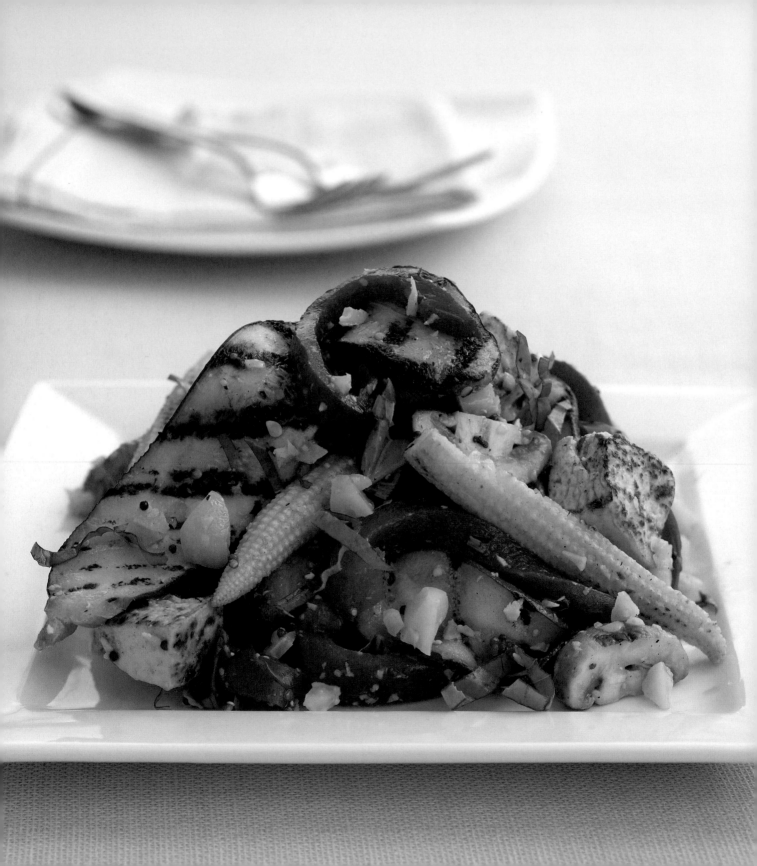

introduction

When our editor, Siobhan Gooley, was working on *The Low GI Diet Revolution*, she kept asking us, "What about me and all those other vegetarians out there?" Well, we said, vegetarians are usually healthier than most people and probably already eat a low glycemic index diet. They also tend to be slimmer and more active, have a reduced risk of diabetes and heart disease, and already know about the benefits of legumes and whole grains and eating plenty of fruit and vegetables. "Not necessarily," said Siobhan. "Vegetarians often have a diet that's high in saturated fat from dairy foods but low in omega-3. And we worry about getting all the nutrients we need for long-term health and well-being, just like everyone else."

So, this book introducing vegetarians and vegans to healthy low GI eating is for Siobhan and everyone following, or interested in eating, a vegetarian or vegan diet. We hope you will find it informative and inspirational in getting your eating habits into shape so you can enjoy the benefits of low GI fare. We show you where you will find the fuels you need to keep your body's metabolism or engine running smoothly, and give plenty of meal ideas and menus for vegetarian and vegan adults, teenagers and children. And, we explain why the glycemic index and low GI carbs matter.

There are 80 mouth-watering recipes packed with nutrition and full of flavor. We have made sure that they are rich in plant protein, good fats, fruit and vegetables and healthy whole grains. We hope that you enjoy trying them as much as we have loved creating them.

Jennie, Kaye, Kate and Philippa

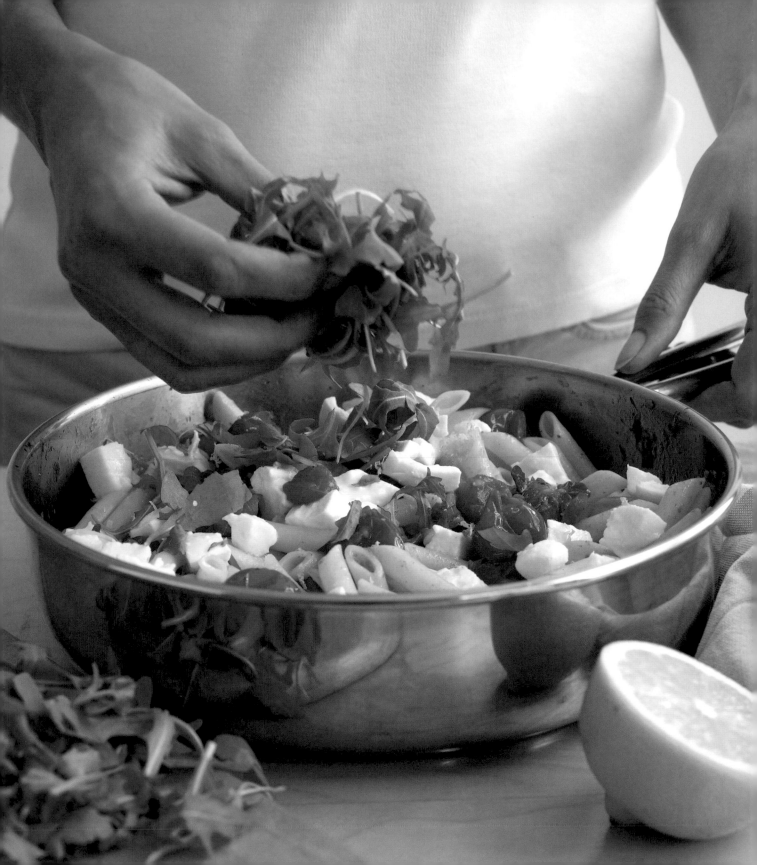

part one

the healthy vegetarian

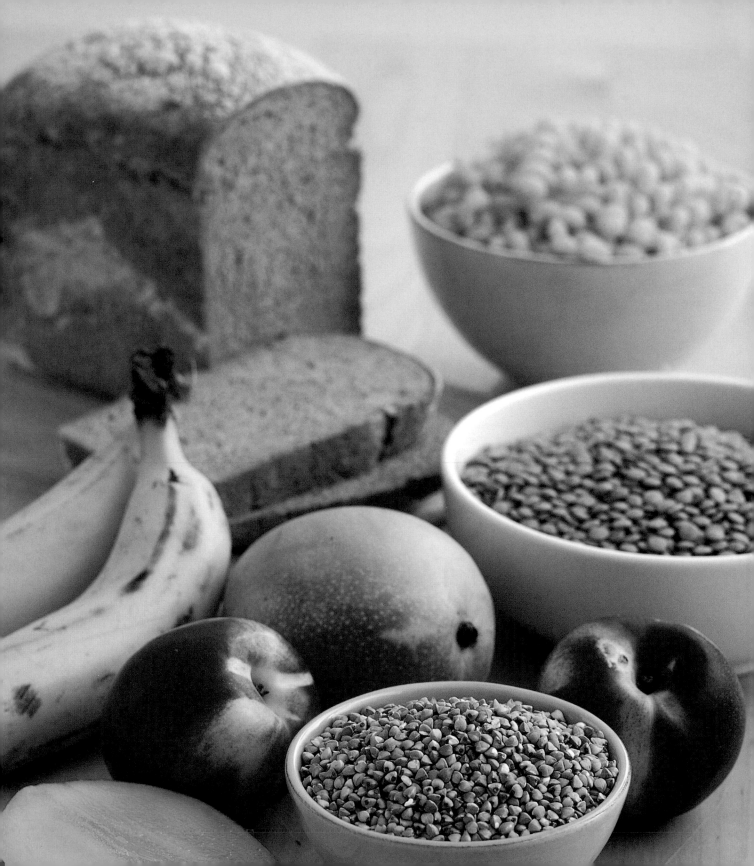

what should I eat?

Building your diet around plant foods such as whole grains, legumes, fruits, vegetables, nuts and seeds gives you all the nutrients you need for long-term health and well-being, along with plenty of protective antioxidants and phytochemicals. Not only that, there's now a wealth of scientific evidence to support the fact that a vegetarian diet can reduce the risk of heart disease, diabetes and cancer.

In this chapter, we answer the perennial "what should I eat?" question by looking at the essential fuels you need to keep your engine running smoothly (protein, carbohydrates and fat)—what they do and where you can find them. We then show you how vegetarians and vegans can get their diet into top shape with all the necessary vitamins and minerals, especially iron, zinc, calcium and vitamin B_{12}.

Protein

We are made of protein—our muscles, bones, skin, hair and virtually every other body part. Protein consists of basic "building blocks" called amino acids. There are 20 different amino acids and they can be found in many of the foods we eat. The body makes some amino acids on its own (non-essential amino acids); but there are eight "essential" amino acids our bodies can't make and we need to get them from food. Because our bodies can't stockpile them from one day to the next as they do fat or carbs, we need a daily supply of protein foods to maintain our body tissues and keep the engine in good repair.

What are the best sources?

It's not necessary to eat red meat, chicken or fish to get enough protein. Plant proteins can provide you with all the essential and non-essential amino acids you need, so long as you eat plenty of legumes (beans, chickpeas and lentils), foods rich in soy protein (such as tofu), cereal grains (especially whole grains), and nuts and seeds. It's even easier if you eat dairy foods and eggs. Following is our checklist of the best sources of protein in a well-balanced vegetarian diet.

Legumes

Whether you buy them dried or canned, beans such as kidney, cannellini, cranberry and haricot beans, or even good old baked beans, are one of nature's nutritional power packs. First, they are a valuable source of protein for vegetarians and vegans—200 g (7 oz) of home-cooked or canned beans, lentils or chickpeas provides an

Eggs

Eggs are not only a great convenience food for quick and easy meals, they provide protein (2 large eggs provide 12 g of protein) plus essential vitamins and minerals, including vitamins A, D, E and B-group vitamins, and iron, phosphorus and zinc. Their cholesterol content is only a concern if you have high blood cholesterol levels and/or your diet is high in saturated fat. Omega-3 enriched eggs can make a significant contribution to the long-chain omega-3 fats—vital to human brain development and function.

average of 15 g of protein, which is why we recommend you eat them every day. Second, they are high in fiber and are an important source of carbs, B vitamins (including folate), minerals such as iron, zinc and magnesium, and potent phytochemicals. They are versatile, too: you can add them to soups and salads, casseroles and stir-fries, use them as a topping or filling, or make them into spreads such as hummus.

Low fat dairy foods and fortified soy alternatives

Just 1 cup (9 fl oz) of skim milk, a 200 g (7 oz) tub of low fat yogurt, or a 30 g (1 oz) piece of low fat cheddar cheese provide almost 10 g of protein along with calcium, and vitamins A, B and D. It's surprising the number of people who think butter, being a dairy food, is a source of calcium. It isn't. Nor is cream or sour cream. They are primarily sources of saturated fat.

Soy beans and soy products

Protein-rich soy beans have long been a staple of Asian diets. Just 200 g (7 oz) of cooked or canned soy beans provides 24 g of protein. They are also rich in fiber, iron, zinc, vitamin B, and phytochemicals. They are higher in fat than other legumes, but the majority of that fat is polyunsaturated. Soy protein has also been found to help lower cholesterol levels in the blood. Soy beans are the basis of a variety of protein-rich products and meat substitutes, including tofu, tempeh, textured vegetable protein (TVP), and vegetarian sausages and burgers.

If you choose not to eat dairy products, soy beverages, cheeses, yogurts and desserts are excellent nutritional equivalents with the added benefits of being low in saturated fat, cholesterol free and rich in phytochemicals. However, soy products are not naturally high in calcium and can still be high in fat, so it is important to look for calcium-fortified varieties and to choose low fat products if watching your weight.

Nuts and seeds

Fill up your protein tank with a handful of nuts—a 30 g (1 oz) serving of most nuts provides around 5 g protein; macadamias and pecans have less. All nuts are among the richest sources of the antioxidants vitamin E and selenium in our diet, but they are high in fat—mainly unsaturated. A small handful makes a healthy snack, a crunchy topping for salads, stir-fries and desserts, or you can add nuts (whole or chopped) to muesli mixes, fillings and stuffings to boost the nutritional benefits. Make sure you choose the unsalted variety and enjoy in moderation—it's always tempting to eat more of these.

Seeds such as sesame (and tahini, a paste of sesame seeds), pumpkin, sunflower and flaxseeds also play a valuable role in the diet, and not just for their protein content. Just 15 g (½ oz) provides about 3–4 g protein along with iron, zinc, essential fatty acids and a range of vitamins, minerals and antioxidants. Add them to mueslis, oatmeal, salads, stir-fries and baking, and mix them together to make a healthy sprinkle.

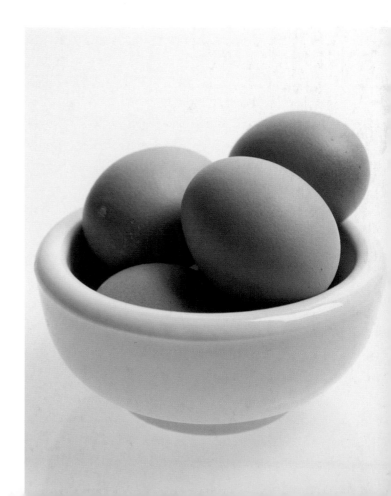

Cereal grains

Grains are the seeds of cereal plants and include barley, buckwheat, bulgur, maize, millet, oats, quinoa, rice, rye, spelt and wheat. Whether you eat them as whole grains (such as brown rice or pearl barley), processed (such as white rice) or as one of the staple foods made from them (bread, breakfast cereals, pasta, noodles and couscous), they play an important role in vegetarian and vegan diets. Did you know that 1 cup (7½ oz) of cooked brown rice provides nearly 6 g of protein, and a slice of mixed-grain bread or 30 g (1 oz) of raw rolled oats around 3 g? They are also the most concentrated sources of carbs in our diet, are low in fat, packed with essential vitamins and minerals, rich in fiber if you eat whole grain varieties, and are the basis for a wide range of convenient and economical meals and snacks. Studies around the world show that eating plenty of whole grains reduces the risk of certain types of cancer, heart disease and type 2 diabetes.

Wheat protein and seitan

Seitan (pronounced *say-tahn*) is sometimes called "wheat meat". It comes from wheat gluten (the protein part of flour) and is an alternative to soy-based meat substitutes such as tofu. A traditional food for Buddhists, it is more like meat than textured vegetable protein (TVP) or mycoprotein (Quorn™), for example. It has a chewy texture and neutral taste and tends to absorb the flavor of the foods you cook it with. Just add it to cooked dishes at the last minute, heating just until it is warmed through. Seitan is sold chilled in tubs or frozen in blocks, chunks, strips, or

Protein and weight loss

There has been a lot in the press about high protein diets being the key to rapid weight loss. It is true that eating protein at each meal will help keep hunger pangs at bay and reduce the urge to snack, but longer term studies have not shown any significant benefits of high protein diets, and there are some concerns about following such an eating plan long term. Your protein intake should always be balanced with a variety of whole grains and other healthy low GI carbs to ensure you're getting all the micronutrients you need.

ground. You will probably have to check the tofu section of health-food or Asian produce stores. You can also buy powdered wheat gluten, which you mix with water for do-it-yourself seitan. But the result doesn't deliver quite the same chewy texture.

Mycoprotein (Quorn™)

Mycoprotein is manufactured from the mold *Fusarium venenatum,* which is grown in large sterile fermentation tanks. Glucose is added (as a food for the fungus), as are various vitamins and minerals (to improve the product's nutrition value). After harvesting, it is heat treated and then mixed with egg whites, which act as a binder (so it's not suitable for vegans). Finally, the product is textured to resemble meat and pressed into a mince or into chunks for home cooking (it can be grilled, sautéed, baked or added to casseroles), or used in ready-prepared meals. Marketed as Quorn™, it is low in saturated fat and a good source of protein (100 g/3½ oz supplies about 12 g of protein), fiber, iron and zinc. You can find it in health-food stores and major supermarket chains mainly in the US, UK, and Europe.

How much protein do you need?

To maintain your body tissues and keep the engine in good repair you need around 40–55 g (1½–2 oz) of protein a day—a lot less than popular weight-loss diets promote, and easily achievable with a well-balanced diet. On average, women need about 45 g of protein a day (more, if they are pregnant or breastfeeding) and men about 55 g. If you are active you may need more, and growing teenagers certainly do as well. In the menu plans (pages 55–67) and recipes (from page 69) you'll see how easy it is to get sufficient protein on a vegetarian or vegan diet.

Protein: the bottom line

- Eat a wide variety of protein foods every day to make sure you get all the essential amino acids you need.
- Stock your pantry with legumes, whole grains (such as grainy breads, muesli, brown rice, pearl barley and rolled oats), nuts and seeds (sesame seeds, tahini and pumpkin seeds). They are good sources of protein and the key nutrients iron and zinc typically sourced from protein-rich foods.

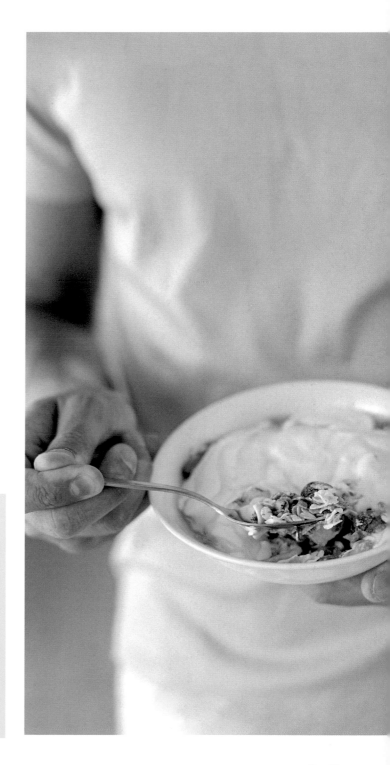

Fats

For vegetarians and non-vegetarians alike, the message is: know your fats. Focus on the good fats and give the bad ones the boot. A low fat diet is not necessarily the only way to eat for overall health or even weight loss. Your body needs a certain amount of good or unsaturated fat—think nuts, seeds, olive oil and avocados—to function properly and thrive. Good fats:

- provide you with essential fatty acids
- help you absorb the fat-soluble vitamins A, D, E and K
- form part of your body's hormones
- provide insulation
- help you absorb some antioxidants from fruit and vegetables
- help to make food taste better.

Your body actually requires some types of fats—called essential fatty acids—which can't be manufactured by your body and so have to be obtained through your diet. The best sources of these for vegetarians are polyunsaturated oils, flaxseeds and flaxseed oil, mustard seed oil, canola oil, nuts and seeds.

The big problem with fat is the amount we eat, sometimes without realizing it. Fat provides lots of calories—more than protein or carbs per gram. The main form in which our bodies store those extra calories is, you guessed it, fat.

It's easy to reduce your fat intake when you know it's there (the most concentrated sources of fat in our diets are butter, margarines and oils). But snack foods, cakes, cookies, potato chips and muffins, regular popcorn or a package of instant noodles all contain a fair bit of fat as well. That's why it's important to read the label. When shopping, look for products low in saturated fat, rather than just low fat products. The saturated fat content should be less than 20 percent of the total fat.

Cheese can be a major source of saturated fat in vegetarian diets—all too often a cheesy dish is the only vegetarian option on the restaurant menu. Most cheese is around 30 percent fat, much of it saturated. So, opt for low fat choices such as ricotta or cottage cheese for your everyday cheese choice, and if you can't live without a regular fix of tasty full fat varieties, check out our tips for making the most of cheese on page 50.

Choose the good fats and oils

- Olive, peanut and canola oils
- Mustard seed, avocado, rice bran and macadamia oils
- Flaxseed oil (can't be heated)
- Soft margarines and spreads made with olive, canola, sunflower or other seed oils
- Avocados, olives
- Soy beans
- Almonds, brazil nuts, cashews, hazelnuts, macadamias, pistachio nuts, peanuts, walnuts, etc.
- Flaxseeds, sunflower seeds, pumpkin seeds, sesame seeds
- Nut and seed spreads such as peanut butter, almond spread or tahini
- Muesli (untoasted).

Give the bad fats the boot

- Full cream (full fat) dairy products—milk, cream, sour cream, cream cheese, cheese, ice cream
- Coconut and palm oils
- Copha, ghee and solid frying oils and margarines
- Potato chips, packaged snacks
- Cakes, cookies, pastries, pies, pizza
- Deep-fried foods—chips, spring rolls, tempura, battered foods.

How much fat do you need?

Not much. Unless you are a very active person, 2–4 servings a day is all you need. One serving is equivalent to:

- 2 teaspoons of monounsaturated or polyunsaturated oil or margarine
- 1 tablespoon of oil-based vinaigrette
- 15 g (½ oz) of nuts
- 40 g (1½ oz) of avocado.

Polyunsaturated fats are made up of omega-3 and omega-6 fats and the balance between these is important for good health.

Since vegetarians tend to consume more omega-6 and less omega-3, focus on including foods that are specifically sources of omega-3, such as walnuts, flaxseeds, soy products or flaxseed oil. When preparing meals, try using a variety of different oils, depending on the dish— a monounsaturated oil such as canola or olive oil is a good idea for cooking, as these oils are both "omega-neutral", meaning they will not worsen the balance of omega-6:omega-3.

Fats: the bottom line

- Focus on the good fats.
- Choose low fat dairy products.
- Be aware of the hidden fats in snack foods.
- Stock your pantry with nuts and seeds that are good sources of omega-3.

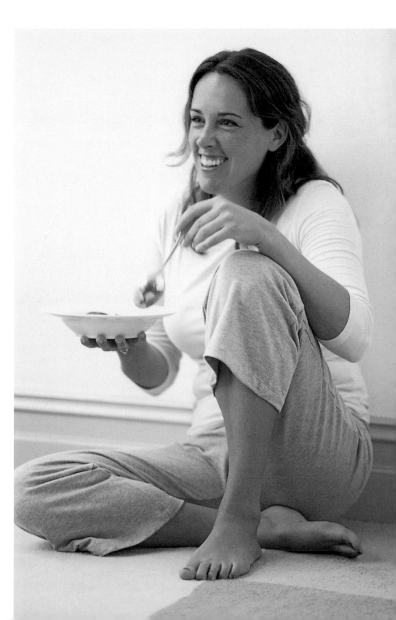

Carbohydrates

Carbohydrates are the mostly widely consumed substances in the world after water. A vital source of energy, it's found in all plants and in its simplest form, glucose is:

- a universal fuel for our bodies
- the only fuel source for our brain, red blood cells and a growing fetus
- the main source of energy for our muscles during strenuous exercise.

Some foods contain a large amount of carbohydrates (cereals, potatoes, sweet potatoes, legumes and corn are good examples), while others, such as string beans, broccoli and salad greens, have only very small amounts of carbohydrates. Breast milk, cow's milk and milk products also contain carbohydrates in the form of milk sugar, or lactose.

What are the best sources?

Vegetarians and vegans generally eat high-carb diets, and that's why carb quality really counts. On page 12 we explain the importance of carb quality in more detail. First of all, let's look at where you can find the good sources of carbohydrates.

Grains

Cereal grains such as barley, buckwheat, bulgur, maize, millet, oats, quinoa, rice, rye, spelt and wheat, and the enormous variety of foods made from them, including bread, breakfast cereals, pasta, noodles and couscous, are the richest sources of carbohydrates. They also provide you with fiber and protein and many vitamins and minerals, especially if you choose whole grain foods.

Each of the following servings will give you between 20–30 g of carbohydrates:

- 2 slices of bread
- 1 cup of breakfast cereal
- ½ cup of rolled oats or muesli
- ½ cup of cooked rice or other small grains such as bulgur or cracked wheat
- 1 cup of cooked pasta, noodles or couscous.

Legumes

These are probably the second-richest source of carbohydrates in a vegetarian diet (1 cup of cooked or canned beans, chickpeas or lentils provides between 20–30 g of carbohydrate), as well as being a major source of protein, vitamin B, iron and zinc.

Vegetables

The higher-carbohydrate vegetables are the starchy ones that grow under the ground—potato, taro, yam and sweet potato (2 small potatoes or half a medium sweet potato, for example, will provide 20–30 g of carbohydrate). If you eat large servings (bigger than 1 cup) then you could consider parsnip, beet, pumpkin, carrot, turnips and peas as additional sources of carbohydrates. Corn, while strictly a grain, is also high in carbohydrates (1 cup of kernels or a cob of corn will provide 20–30 g of carbohydrate). Most other vegetables are low in carbohydrates, but are often valuable sources of vitamins and minerals along with protective antioxidants.

Fruit

A high fruit and vegetable intake has been consistently linked with better health (as have vegetarian diets)—perhaps because fruits and vegetables are packed with antioxidants. Fruit will also contribute to your carbohydrate intake (in the form of fruit sugars) but doesn't provide nearly as much carbohydrate as the cereal grains. Dried fruits are an exception, with many being as high in carbohydrate as cereal grains (a 30 g/1 oz serving provides between 10–20 g of carbohydrate), and they are also a concentrated source of many vitamins and minerals.

Low fat dairy foods and soy alternatives

Don't overlook calcium-rich dairy foods as a source of carbohydrate in the form of lactose. Consuming 1 cup (9 fl oz) of low fat or skim milk will provide you with about 12 g of carbohydrate. Soy beverages do not contain lactose but generally contain the sugar sucrose, and 1 cup contains around 15 g of carbohydrate. Look for the low fat, calcium-enriched varieties. Dairy products including yogurt, custard and ice cream (and the soy equivalents) are also good sources of carbohydrate, but not cheese (the lactose is removed from whey during the cheese manufacturing process).

How much carbohydrate do you need?

Vegetarian and vegan diets tend to be high in carbs (and fiber too) because they are plant-based. The number of calories, and hence the amount of carbohydrate you eat, will vary with your weight and activity levels.

- If you are an active person with average energy requirements you'll need around 275 g (10 oz) of carbohydrate a day to keep that engine humming along. How do you get it? Well, 275 g (10 oz) is equal to ½ cup of muesli, 4 slices of bread, 2 cups of cooked pasta, 1 cup of cooked or canned legumes, 3 servings of fruit and 2 servings of milk/soy milk or yogurt. And you haven't even added in the day's vegetables.

- If you are trying to lose weight and are on a calorie diet (i.e., a small eater on around 1200 calories a day), about 165 g of carbohydrate a day should be sufficient to maintain your normal activity levels. That's equal to ½ cup muesli, 2 slices of bread, 1 cup of cooked pasta, 1 cup of cooked or canned legumes, 2 servings of fruit and 2 servings of milk/soy milk or yogurt. And again, you haven't started on the vegetables.

But in the end, the choice of how much carbohydrate you eat a day—moderate or high—is yours. What really matters is the type or source of the carbohydrate. Remember we said earlier that quality counts; it is just as important as the amount. Here's why.

How your body revs on carbs

When you eat foods such as bread, cereals and fruit, your body converts them into a sugar called glucose during digestion. This glucose is absorbed from your intestine into your bloodstream and becomes the fuel that circulates around your body. As the level of blood glucose rises after you have eaten a meal, your pancreas gets the message to release a powerful hormone called insulin. Insulin drives glucose out of your blood and into the cells. Once inside, glucose will be channeled into various pathways simultaneously—it will be used as an immediate source of energy or converted to glycogen (a storage form of glucose), or converted into fat. Insulin also turns off the use of fat as the cell's energy source. For this reason, lowering your insulin levels is beneficial to losing weight, and is one of the secrets to lifelong health. In the next chapter we explain how understanding the GI of foods helps you choose not only the right amount of carbohydrate, but also the right type for your long-term health and well-being.

The GI—today's dietary power tool

Not all carbs are created equal. In fact, they can behave quite differently in our bodies. The glycemic index, or GI, is how we describe this difference. It ranks carbs (sugars and starches) according to their effect on blood glucose levels. After testing hundreds of foods around the world, researchers have now found that foods with a low GI will have less of an effect on our blood glucose levels than foods with a high GI. High GI foods tend to cause spikes in our glucose levels, whereas low GI foods cause gentle rises.

- High GI foods such as white bread, potatoes, jelly beans and corn flakes are converted to glucose quickly in your body.
- Low GI foods such as rolled oats, apples, pasta and yogurt are converted to glucose slowly in your body.

Switching to eating predominantly low GI carbs that slowly trickle glucose into your bloodstream keeps your energy levels perfectly balanced and means you will feel fuller for longer between meals. The idea is to replace highly refined carbs

Carbs: the bottom line

To ensure that you are eating enough carbohydrate and the right kind, you should eat:

- fruits or vegetables at every meal, or for snacks
- at least one low GI food at each meal
- lots of fiber-rich whole grains.

GI values

Low GI = 55 or less
Medium GI = 56 to 69
High GI = 70 or more
To check out the GI of your favorite carbs visit:
www.glycemicindex.com

such as white bread, sugary sweets and rice crispies with less processed ones such as whole grain bread, pasta, beans, fruit and vegetables. We like to say that your body should do the food processing, not the manufacturer.

Choosing low GI carbs will not only promote weight control, it will reduce blood glucose and insulin levels throughout the day, increase your sense of feeling full and satisfied, and provide fibre and a rich supply of micronutrients, including zinc, calcium and magnesium.

The key to understanding GI is the rate of digestion

Foods containing carbs that break down quickly during digestion have the highest GI value. The blood glucose response is fast and high (in other words, the glucose in the bloodstream increases rapidly). Conversely, foods that contain carbs which break down slowly, releasing glucose gradually into the bloodstream, have low GI values.

For most people, the foods with a low GI have advantages over those with high GI values. This is especially true for those people trying to prevent heart disease and type 2 diabetes.

The higher the GI, the higher the blood glucose levels after you have eaten the food. Instant white rice (GI of 87) and baked potatoes (GI of 85) have very high GIs, meaning their effect on blood glucose levels is almost as high as that of an equal amount of pure glucose (yes, you read it correctly).

How low GI foods can help with losing weight

- They fill you up and keep you satisfied longer than their high GI counterparts.
- They reduce insulin levels and help you burn more body fat and less muscle, so that your metabolic rate is higher.

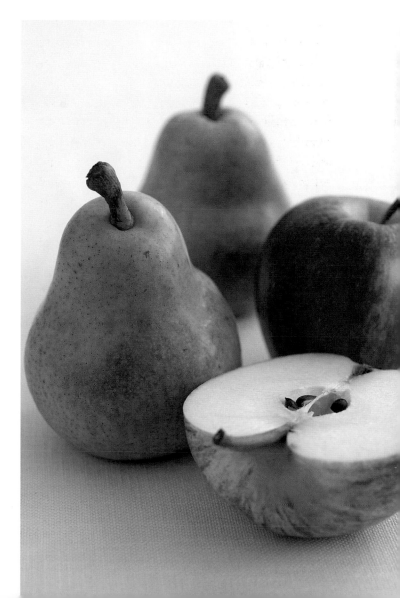

Are you eating enough fiber?

Many low GI foods are good sources of dietary fiber, which is a terrific bonus since we need about 30 g of fiber a day for good bowel health. Filling, high-fiber foods can also help you maintain a healthy weight by reducing hunger pangs.

Dietary fiber only comes from plant foods—it is found in the outer bran layers of grains (corn, oats, wheat and rice and in foods containing these grains), fruit, vegetables, nuts and legumes (dried beans, peas and lentils). There are two types of fiber—soluble and insoluble.

- *Soluble fibers* are the gel, gum and often jelly-like components of apples, oats and legumes. By slowing down the time it takes for food to pass through the stomach and small intestine, soluble fiber can lower the glycemic response to a food. Good sources include: oatmeal, oat bran, nuts and seeds, legumes (beans, peas and lentils), apples, pears, strawberries and blueberries.

- *Insoluble fibers* are dry and bran-like, and are commonly called roughage. All cereal grains and products that retain the outer coat of the grain they are made from are sources of insoluble fiber, e.g. wholemeal bread and All-Bran®, but not all foods containing insoluble fiber are low GI. Insoluble fibers will only lower the GI of a food when they exist in their original, intact form, for example in whole grains of wheat. Here they act as a physical barrier, delaying access of digestive enzymes and water to the starch within the cereal grain.

Good sources include: whole grains, whole wheat breads, barley, couscous, brown rice, bulgur, wheat bran, seeds, and most vegetables.

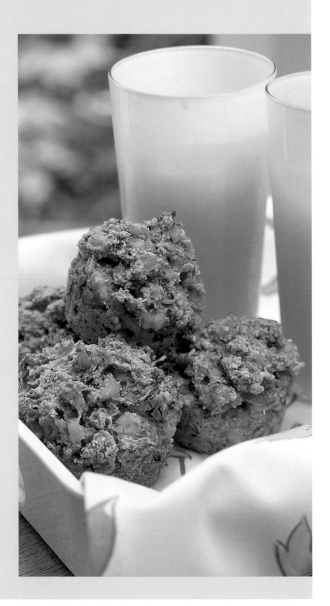

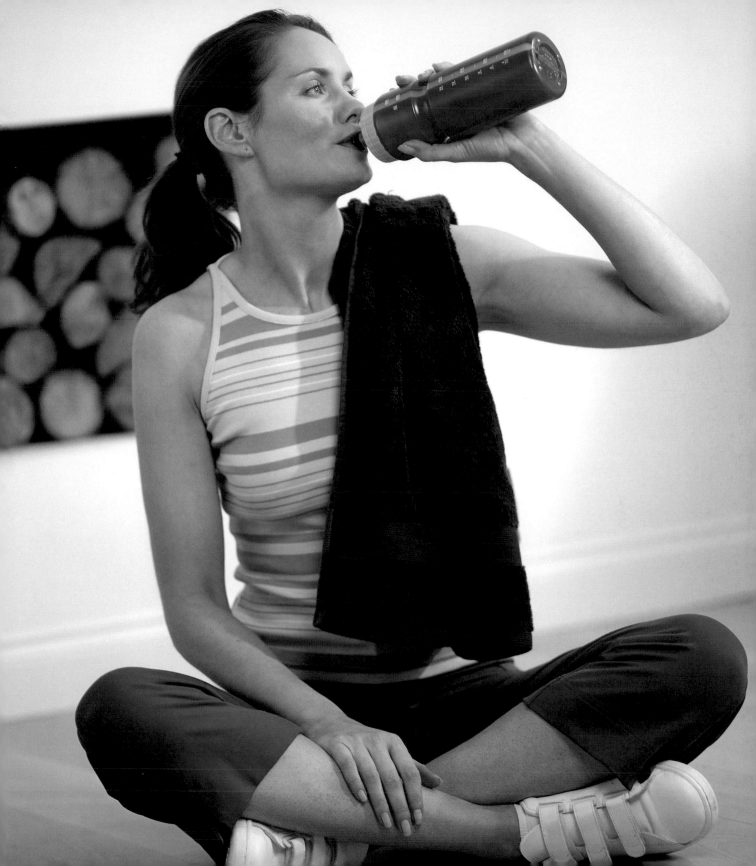

What about vitamins and minerals?

While there are some nutrients which can be more difficult to obtain in vegetarian and vegan diets, with a little knowledge of the best plant sources and tricks to enhance their absorption by the body, you can get all the essential nutrients you need. Here we outline the functions and best sources of iron, zinc, calcium and B_{12}. To give you an idea how much iron, zinc and calcium you need each day, we have included the latest nutrient requirements from the National Health and Medical Research Council, which applies to both Australia and New Zealand. The US recommended nutrient intakes for these minerals are similar.

Iron

We need iron in our diet and many of us (especially women) need more than we are currently getting. This essential mineral plays a vital role in:

- forming hemoglobin, which transports oxygen around the body
- assisting in energy-producing chemical reactions.

When it comes to iron, you need to know that there are two types and there is a difference.

- Heme iron is found in animal foods such as meat, chicken, fish and offal.
- Non-heme iron is found in eggs and plant foods such as legumes, cereal grains, nuts, seeds, dark-green leafy vegetables and dried fruit.

The difference matters because humans can absorb heme iron much more readily than non-heme iron. In fact, the body absorbs around 15–25 percent of heme iron from animal sources, but only around 2–5 percent of non-heme iron from plant sources. However, you can increase the absorption of non-heme iron if you eat or drink vitamin C-rich fruits and vegetables at the same meal. That's why it's a good idea to have a glass of orange juice with your breakfast cereal or a good portion of salad on your whole grain sandwich.

What are the best sources?

Legumes

Legumes play a star role in a healthy low GI diet and they top the list as a source of iron for vegetarians and vegans—1 cup of cooked beans, chickpeas or lentils provides nearly 4 mg of iron and just ½ cup of baked beans provides 2.2 mg.

The phytate factor

Some natural compounds in plants such as phytates and oxalates (found in spinach, rhubarb, chard and beet greens), as well as tannins in tea and coffee, can inhibit iron absorption. This is because they bind and hold iron so your body can't absorb it properly. Excessive calcium-rich foods and supplements can also inhibit iron absorption if you have them at the same meal. However, eating a wide variety of foods over the day should ensure that the benefits of vitamin C intake override the phytate effect.

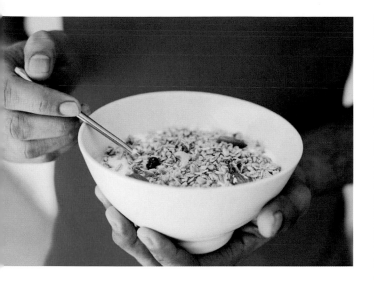

Soy products

Soy products are another source of iron—100 g (3½ oz) of tempeh or 200 g (7 oz) of firm tofu provide more than 2 g iron.

Cereal grains

Whole grains are a good source of iron, along with fortified breakfast cereals (look for low GI ones), wheat germ, grainy breads, rolled oats, brown rice and natural muesli. To start the day, an average 30 g (1 oz) serving of a commercial breakfast cereal delivers 3 mg of iron, while 2 slices of whole grain or wholemeal bread for a lunchtime sandwich provide 1.2 mg. For dinner, serve your meal with some brown rice (1 cup of cooked rice provides 0.9 mg).

Nuts and seeds

If you are looking for little ways to up your daily iron intake, don't underestimate the power of a handful or nuts or seeds. A handful (30 g/1 oz)

What vegetarians need to know about iron

Anemia caused by iron deficiency can be a nutritional issue for vegetarians, and, in particular, for women. Iron deficiency can make you more vulnerable to catching colds and other infections, so it's important to keep your iron intake up.

The primary function of iron is to transport oxygen to all the organs, muscles and tissues in the body. So, if you often feel overtired, weak, headache-prone or have trouble doing exercise, it may be a good idea to get your doctor to test your iron levels.

It is recommended that all vegetarians try to include some plant-based sources of iron at every meal. These include:

- tofu
- legumes
- whole grain cereals
- green leafy vegetables such as broccoli or spinach
- nuts
- dried fruits
- eggs
- seeds, such as sunflower seeds.

of pistachios adds 4 g of iron. Other nuts and seeds that are good sources of iron are almonds, cashews, macadamias, pecans, pine nuts, walnuts and sunflower seeds. Or simply top your toast with a tablespoon of peanut butter or other nut spreads.

Vegetables

The best vegetable sources of iron are the dark-green leafy vegetables, including broccoli (just ½ cup gives 1 mg of iron), Asian greens, kale and spinach.

Fruit

Dried fruits are a good source of iron. A few apricots (5 or 6 halves) provide 0.7 g of iron. Other dried fruits that are useful sources or iron are figs, prunes, dates and raisins. Just ⅔ cup (5½ fl oz) of prune juice provides 2.5 g of iron.

Eggs

That boiled egg for breakfast has 1.1 g of iron. But the iron is in the yolk, so don't be tempted by those egg-white omelets offered on the menu in trendy cafés these days.

How much iron do you need?

Women need two to three times more iron than men because of menstruation and pregnancy. Unless you have been diagnosed as having an iron deficiency by your doctor, it is best not to take iron supplements simply because you are vegetarian or vegan. Most vegetarians should be able to obtain an adequate iron intake if they eat a well-balanced diet.

Taking too much iron can cause iron overload in some people, so if you choose to take a supplement, have your iron levels tested regularly.

Iron: the bottom line

- Eat legumes, tofu, dark-green leafy vegetables and whole grains regularly.
- Include a vitamin C-rich fruit or vegetable at each meal.
- Limit your intake of tea and coffee and drink them between meals rather than with meals.

Iron	Milligrams per day
Men	8
Women	8–18
Pregnant women	27

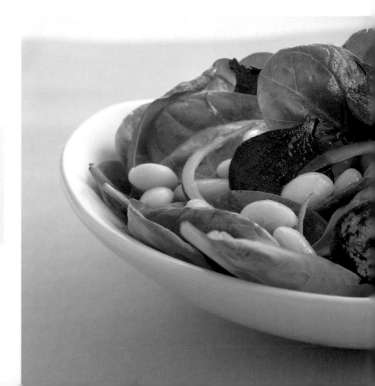

Zinc

We need zinc for a healthy immune system. It's a key player in fighting infections and helping cuts and wounds to heal. Life without zinc would not be quite so enjoyable—we absolutely have to have it to help us smell, taste and see.

Only about 20 percent of the zinc from the food we eat is actually absorbed by the body. The richest sources are animal foods, and they are the best absorbed sources too. Vegetarians can, however, get all the zinc they need from plant sources, but it's important to be aware that, as with iron, the phytate factor can come into play and inhibit the absorption of zinc.

What are the best sources?

If you eat a well-balanced diet as we have outlined, you are unlikely to run low on zinc. Here are some of the best sources.

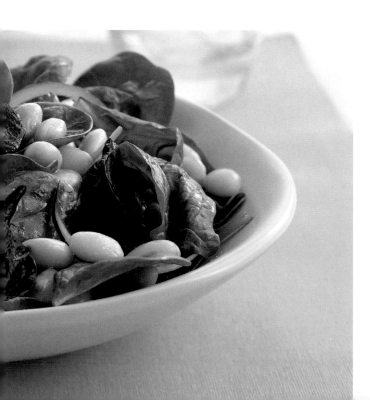

Dairy foods
Low fat milk, yogurt and cheese.

Legumes
Beans, chickpeas, lentils and dhal.

Nuts
Almonds, brazil nuts, cashews and peanuts.

Seeds
Sesame seeds, tahini, and especially pumpkin seeds, which provide one of the most concentrated sources of zinc for vegetarians.

Whole grain cereals
The outer husk of whole grains contains zinc, but it's lost when those products are refined, so opt for grainy breads, muesli and whole cereal grains like brown rice or pearl barley and rolled oats.

How much zinc do you need?

Zinc	Milligrams per day
Men	14
Women	8
Pregnant women	11

Zinc: the bottom line
- Eat legumes, tofu, nuts, seeds and whole grains regularly.

Calcium

The key to strong, healthy bones is making sure you have plenty of calcium in your diet. Milk, cheese, yogurt, ice cream, buttermilk and custard, as well as calcium-fortified soy products, are among the richest sources, and for most vegetarians the easiest way to get the calcium you need. By replacing full fat dairy foods with reduced fat, low fat or fat-free versions, you will reduce your saturated fat intake.

Calcium is the most abundant mineral in our bodies. It builds our bones and teeth and is involved in muscle contraction and relaxation, blood clotting, nerve function and regulation of blood pressure. If we don't get enough calcium in our diet, our bodies will draw it out of our bones. Over a period of time, this can lead to osteoporosis, loss of height, curvature of the spine and periodontal disease, which attacks the bones supporting our teeth. We build our maximum bone strength by about 20 years of age. From our early thirties, bone calcium starts decreasing, but an adequate calcium intake, among other things, can help slow the decline.

Studies are now showing that calcium:

- can help lower high blood pressure
- may protect against some cancers
- can favorably influence blood fat levels and reduce the risk of stroke
- can reduce the risk of kidney stones
- may assist in weight regulation.

As with iron and zinc, the amount of calcium your body absorbs from food is something of a balancing act. The phytic acid found in bran, cereals and raw vegetables can inhibit calcium absorption. So choose whole grain breads and cereals rather than adding bran, and make sure each day that you have some of your vegetables cooked. Eating more salt in your diet significantly increases the amount of calcium you excrete, as does eating more animal protein.

Here are our tips to help you maximize your calcium absorption:

- Eat plenty of calcium-rich foods.
- Eat more soy foods—soy protein and the naturally occurring isoflavones may help preserve bone mass; this is particularly important for women in their middle and older years.
- Limit your salt intake.
- Limit your caffeine intake (tea, coffee, cola and "high energy" drinks).
- Make sure that you get enough vitamin D— as little as 10 minutes a day of natural sunlight on the skin of the face, forearms and hands.

What are the best sources?
Dairy foods

Milk and yogurt are key sources of calcium, providing 300 mg of calcium or more per serving, and even more if they have been calcium enriched. A serving consists of 1 cup (9 fl oz) of low fat milk or 200 g (7 oz/1 tub) of low fat yogurt. A 30 g (1 oz) piece of cheddar cheese will provide 230 mg of calcium, and a couple of tablespoons of parmesan grated over your dinner will add 150 mg to your calcium intake. But keep moderation in mind, as these foods are also sources of saturated fat. Cream and butter are not good sources of calcium.

Soy products

If you eat only plant foods or want to avoid dairy products, you may turn to soy beverages, yogurts and desserts as an alternative. Soy products are not naturally high in calcium, so look for calcium-fortified products if you are relying on them as a source of calcium. If you are watching your weight you should choose low fat varieties— 1 cup (9 fl oz) of fortified soy milk has at least 300 mg of calcium.

Tofu

Choose a variety that is set with calcium—100 g (3½ oz) of firm tofu provides 160 mg of calcium. Soft tofu provides about half that, and silken tofu a mere 15 mg of calcium.

Nuts and seeds

A 30 g (1 oz) handful of almonds provides 70 mg of calcium, brazil nuts 55 mg, pistachio nuts 40 mg and walnuts 30 mg. When it comes to seeds, the star performer is unhulled tahini paste, with 1 tablespoon providing 80 mg. Pumpkin, sunflower and sesame seeds are also good sources of calcium.

Fruit

Dried figs are a particularly good source. Two whole dried figs provide 50–150 mg of calcium.

Vegetables

The calcium in the following vegetables is particularly well absorbed: dark-green leafy vegetables, including broccoli; Asian greens like bok choy; kale, collard greens and salad greens such as mesclun. Around ½ cup of greens will provide 50–150 mg of calcium.

How much calcium do you need?

Aim to eat or drink at least two servings of calcium-rich food per day to make sure you meet your calcium needs. It is especially important for pregnant and breastfeeding women and growing children and teenagers to have plenty of calcium in their diets.

Calcium	Milligrams per day
Men (19–50)	1000
Men 50+	1300
Women, 19–50	1000
Women, 50+	1300
Pregnant women	1100 (last trimester)
Teenagers (12-18)	1300
Children (9–11)	1000
Children (4–8)	700

Calcium: the bottom line

- Eat a variety of calcium-rich foods including dairy products or calcium-fortified alternatives.
- Eat more soy foods.
- Include other plant-based sources of calcium regularly in the diet.

What about iodine?

Iodine is a trace element that's vital for our normal development and metabolism. A deficiency can cause goiter (enlargement of the thyroid gland) and impair brain development. In fact, iodine deficiency is the most common cause of preventable mental deficiencies in the world. We only need a small amount of iodine—a teaspoon is a lifetime's supply—but because the body can't store it for long periods we need a little often.

Most of us get all the iodine we need from milk, eggs or by using iodized salt. But some vegetarians and vegans can be at risk of an inadequate iodine intake. It is especially important for pregnant women, as inadequate intake can affect the baby's developing brain. Other good sources of iodine include sea vegetables (seaweeds such as kelp and nori). Sea salt is not a source of iodine.

Vitamin B_{12} (cobalamin)

Vitamin B_{12} is an essential vitamin and the only one that can cause problems for vegetarians, especially vegans, as it is not naturally found in plant foods.

We need B_{12} to form red blood cells and maintain a healthy nervous system. B_{12} deficiency can cause a type of anemia (called megaloblastic anemia), the first symptoms of which are unusual tiredness, difficulty in breathing and dizziness, and can lead to irreversible nerve and brain damage. This is particularly significant for infants, children and women who are pregnant or breastfeeding, as newborn babies have very little of their own stores of vitamin B_{12} and rely on obtaining this from their mothers' breast milk.

B_{12} is found in red meat, offal, poultry and seafood, as well as milk, yogurt, eggs and cheese. The B_{12} is made by bacteria in the large intestine of animals, and is transferred into the animal's meat or milk.

Plant foods including mushrooms, tempeh, miso and sea vegetables are often reported to provide some vitamin B_{12} due to contamination by bacteria. However, any B_{12} they contain is likely to be in a form that the body can't use and may actually prevent the absorption of proper B_{12}.

The only reliable source of B_{12} for vegans is fortified foods or supplements. You will need to read the labels carefully because the amount of B_{12} varies significantly from product to product. B_{12} is best absorbed in small amounts, so ideally you should aim to eat fortified foods two to three times daily.

What are the best sources?

Dairy foods
Low fat milk and cheese. Yogurt is not a good source, as much of the B_{12} is destroyed during the fermentation process.

Eggs
One egg gives 10 percent of the daily requirements of B_{12}.

B_{12} fortified foods
Yeast extracts, veggie burger mixes, textured vegetable protein (TVP), soy milks and breakfast cereals can be fortified with B_{12}. Check the label.

How much B_{12} do you need?
We only need minute amounts of B_{12}, but as you can see this essential vitamin is not found in many foods that vegans eat. If you don't eat eggs, dairy products or foods fortified with vitamin B_{12} then you will need to take a vitamin B_{12} supplement—talk to your doctor or dietitian about how much you need.

Vitamin B_{12}: the bottom line
- Select a variety of foods every day, including eggs, dairy products and B_{12}-fortified foods.
- If you don't eat these foods regularly, you will need to take a B_{12} supplement.

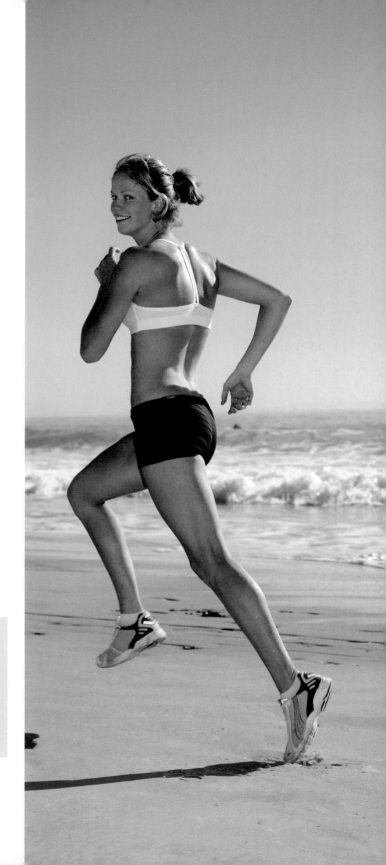

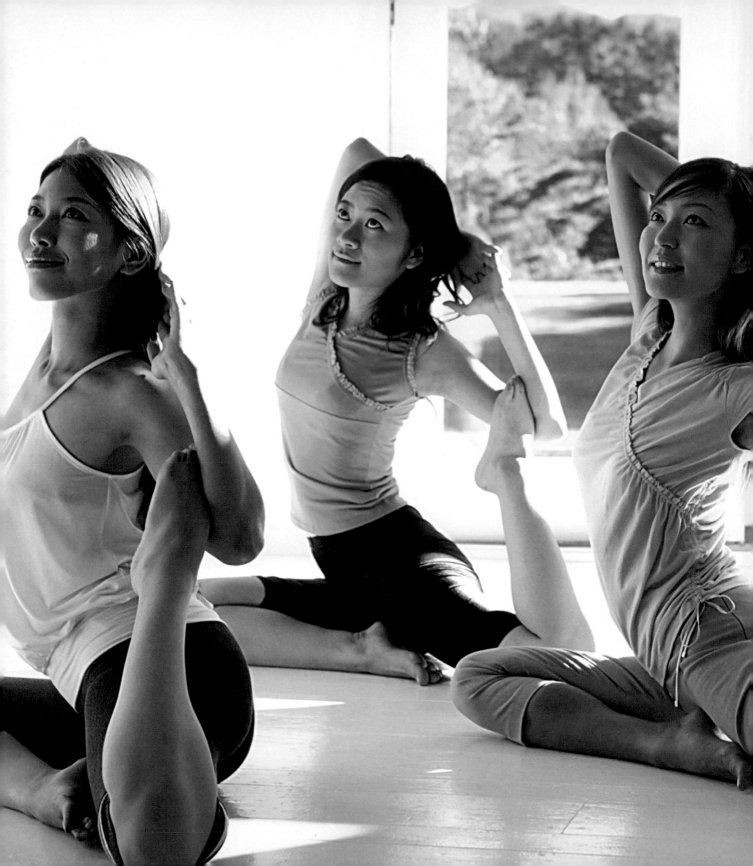

why choose low GI carbs?

Many vegetarians and vegans eat a diet high in carbohydrates, and that's why it's really important to choose the right type of carbs. How can you do this? Well, understanding the GI of foods helps you choose both the right amount of carbohydrate and the right type of carbohydrate for your long-term health and well-being. In this chapter we show you how low GI carbs can make a real difference when it comes to diabetes risk, heart health, weight loss and more.

These days, with such a high proportion of what we eat coming from convenience or take-out foods, our diet tends to be dominated by highly processed and refined high GI carbs—white bread, cookies, light crispy cereals, crackers, potato chips, doughnuts, cakes, and so on.

Eating more of these refined carbs means we are eating fewer traditional starchy foods such as truly whole grain bread (e.g. pumpernickel), fruit, oatmeal, cracked wheat, bulgur, barley, dried peas, beans and lentils. These low GI foods are not only digested more slowly, they are also more micronutrient dense than their counterparts.

Eating a lot of high GI foods can be detrimental to your health because it pushes your body to extremes. This is especially true if you are overweight and sedentary. In the same way that the stormwater pipes of a city are pushed to the limit after a heavy downpour, your body's glucose-response mechanisms are stretched after a load of quickly digested carbs.

What we need to do is replace highly refined starchy carbohydrate foods like most breads, processed breakfast cereals, biscuits, crackers and "instant" meals with less processed carbohydrates in their natural state of whole cereal grains, fruits, legumes and vegetables. Eating more low GI carbs:

- reduces your insulin levels
- lowers your cholesterol levels
- helps control your appetite
- halves your risk of heart disease and diabetes
- means you are eating foods closer to the way nature intended.

For almost everyone, foods with a low GI have advantages over those with high GI values. This is especially true for those people trying to prevent the metabolic syndrome and atherosclerosis (hardening of the arteries).

Why the rate of digestion matters for your health

The type of carbohydrate you eat determines your body's blood glucose response and also determines the levels of insulin in your blood for many hours after eating. High insulin levels caused by eating foods with a high GI are undesirable. In the long term, they promote high blood fat, high blood glucose, high blood pressure and increase the risk of heart attack. Because of this, lowering the GI of your diet is significant in the long-term prevention of heart disease and in improving your overall health.

Diabetes

Did you realize that the higher the GI of your diet, the greater your risk of diabetes? An Australian study of 31,000 people over 10 years found that those who had the highest GI diets were more likely to develop diabetes. In fact, they found that consumption of *white bread* (not sugar!) was most strongly related to the incidence of diabetes.

As we explained earlier, foods with a high GI are digested quickly and cause a rapid rise in blood glucose, and an outpouring of insulin (the hormone that removes glucose from the blood and stores it in cells). If you're eating high GI meals all the time you end up with chronically high insulin levels, which eventually leads to insulin resistance. This means the cells that normally respond to insulin become insensitive to it, so your body thinks it has to make even more insulin to do the job.

All too often, type 2 diabetes is only diagnosed once the pancreas (which produces insulin) is absolutely worn out and cannot maintain sufficient insulin production to normalize blood glucose. Before you get to that point, eating a moderately high carbohydrate, low GI diet can actually improve the function of your pancreas and improve glycemic control, and can therefore prevent the onset of type 2 diabetes.

In an eight-year study of thousands of people in the United States, researchers found that those who ate a high GI diet were almost twice as likely to develop type 2 diabetes. The effect was most pronounced in those people with low levels of physical activity.

In the United States over the past 100 years, the prevalence of obesity and type 2 diabetes has increased in direct proportion to the consumption of refined carbohydrate.

When it comes to diabetes, following a low GI diet can be as effective in lowering your blood glucose as taking diabetes tablets. A scientific analysis of 14 different studies from around the world of people with diabetes showed that low GI diets improved glycemic control significantly more than high GI or conventional diets. Improved glycemic control can prevent the onset and progression of diabetes complications.

On a day-to-day basis, low GI foods can minimize the peaks and valleys in blood glucose that make life so difficult when you have diabetes. Since they are slowly digested and absorbed, low GI foods reduce insulin demand—lessening the strain on the struggling pancreas of a person with type 2 diabetes and potentially lowering insulin requirements for those with type 1 diabetes. Lower insulin levels have the added benefit of reducing the risk of large blood vessel damage, lessening the chance of developing heart disease.

Heart health

These days, most of us are well aware of the importance of cutting back on saturated fat and choosing the "good fats" for heart health. Research on the GI shows that the type of carbohydrate you eat determines your blood glucose response and the levels of insulin in your blood for many hours after you have had a meal or snack. We now know that the higher the GI of your diet the greater your risk of heart disease. A high level of glucose in the blood means:

- more glucose moves into cells lining the arteries, which causes inflammation, thickening and stiffening of artery walls, so the blood vessels lose their elasticity
- highly reactive, charged particles called "free radicals" (like "sparks") are formed, and these destroy the machinery inside the cell, eventually causing the cell to wither and die
- glucose sticks to cholesterol in the blood, which promotes the formation of fatty plaque and prevents the body from breaking down excess cholesterol

- higher levels of insulin are present, which raises blood pressure and blood fats while suppressing "good" (HDL) cholesterol levels.

A diet rich in slowly digested, low GI carbs, on the other hand, along with regular exercise, will reduce your risk of heart disease. By lowering your blood glucose after meals and reducing high insulin levels, you'll have:
- healthier blood vessels that are more elastic, dilate more easily and aid blood flow
- thinner blood and improved blood flow
- more potential for weight loss and therefore less pressure on the heart
- better blood fats—more of the good cholesterol and less of the bad.

In practical terms this means that eating more fruit and vegetables, whole grains, legumes (including beans, chickpeas and lentils) and low fat dairy foods will reduce your risk of heart disease.

Weight loss

There is no doubt that reducing portion sizes and eating fewer calories will lead to weight loss. These days, we are eating less fat but getting fatter. Instead of eating fewer calories we are eating more, especially in the form of high GI refined starches and sugars. The real solution to both weight loss and weight maintenance is to be choosy about the type of carbs you eat. Here are some reasons why:
- Eating high GI carbs causes a surge of glucose in the blood. Although the body

needs glucose it doesn't need this much all in one hit, so it secretes insulin to move the glucose out of the blood and store it in the cells. This drives blood glucose levels down and directs all incoming food to storage—glucose to glycogen and fat, and fats to fat storage.
- The action of insulin means blood glucose levels begin to decline rapidly.
- The brain detects falling blood glucose and, because it relies solely on glucose to keep us alive, it sends out hunger signals.
- The body would normally respond by releasing stored glucose for energy, but if insulin levels remain elevated (as they do in insulin resistance), the release of stored fuel is inhibited.
- Low levels of fuel and high levels of insulin can then trigger the release of stress

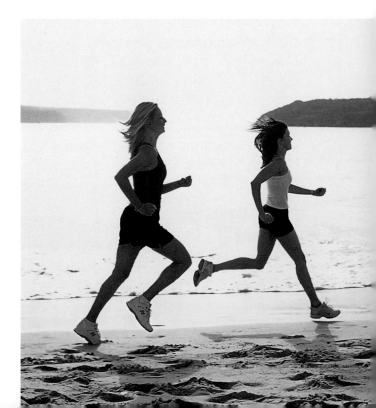

hormones such as adrenaline, which scour the blood for more glucose. This can translate to hunger, light-headedness and feeling shaky. The only way to relieve the state of hunger is with another snack.

Why low GI carbs can help

If you feel hungry all the time, here's how and why low GI foods can help you turn off the switch.

- Low GI foods are rich in carbohydrate— a far superior appetite-suppressant than fat.
- Many low GI foods are less processed, which means they require more chewing— helping to signal satiety to your brain.
- Low GI foods often come in the company of fiber, so they create a greater feeling of fullness in your stomach.
- Low GI foods are more slowly digested, which means they stay in your intestines for longer, keeping you feeling satisfied.
- Low GI foods trickle glucose into your bloodstream slowly, helping you avoid the roller coaster ride in blood glucose levels (a cycle of "sugar highs" followed by "sugar lows").
- Low GI foods help overcome the body's natural tendency to slow down calorie burning (metabolic rate) while dieting.

PCOS

Polycystic ovarian syndrome (PCOS) is thought to affect 5–10 percent of women in developed countries. Characteristics of the syndrome can include irregular periods, infertility, heavy body hair growth, acne, excess weight gain and difficulties in losing weight, but in many women it goes undiagnosed because the symptoms may be subtle, such as faint facial hair. Women with PCOS are also at higher risk of developing diabetes and cardiovascular disease.

Insulin resistance—where the body resists the normal actions of the hormone insulin—is at the root of PCOS. To overcome insulin resistance the body secretes more insulin than normal. Among other effects, this leads to a multiplication of cells in the ovaries, causing a host of hormonal imbalances.

The problem of insulin resistance

Elevations in blood glucose after eating high GI foods are followed by elevations in insulin. When insulin levels are frequently raised, the cells that usually respond to insulin become resistant to its signals. This means that glucose hangs around in the bloodstream at higher-than-normal concentrations, where it can damage cells.

A low GI diet is invaluable in the management of insulin resistance because it will result in lower blood glucose levels after meals, and thereby reduce the demand for insulin. This also has the benefit of assisting appetite control and improving weight loss.

Managing the symptoms of PCOS

To manage PCOS symptoms effectively you need to take charge of your health by managing your weight (body fat), making the change to low GI eating and building more activity into your life. The benefits will include:

- improving PCOS symptoms
- achieving and maintaining healthy weight
- controlling blood glucose and insulin levels
- boosting fertility
- gaining control and quality of life
- reducing your risk of developing diabetes
- reducing your risk of developing heart disease.

If you have PCOS, it is essential to eat in a way that helps to control your insulin levels. This means eating small, regular meals and snacks spread throughout the day, and choosing low GI carbs.

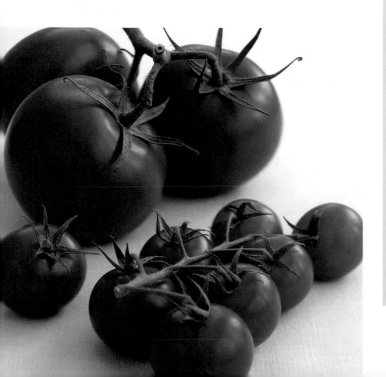

Frequently Asked Questions

Are sugary foods all high GI?

No. This is one of the most widely perpetuated myths, even by so-called proponents of the GI—the sweeter it is the more it spikes your blood glucose. Long-held beliefs are hard to shift. In the recipes you'll discover many deliciously sweet, healthy, low GI foods, from low fat ice cream and chocolate milk to floral honey and fresh fruit.

Should I add up the GI each day?

No. Your diet is not the sum of the GIs, but the average of all the foods you eat. To be precise, you need to take account of how much carbohydrate each food contributes, as well as its GI. We prefer simply to categorize foods as low, medium or high GI and use the "this for that" approach. We find that people who consistently substitute high with low GI foods in their everyday meals and snacks reduce the overall GI of their diet, gain better blood glucose control and lose weight.

Should I avoid all high GI foods?

No. There is no need to eat only low GI foods. While you will benefit from eating low GI carbs at each meal, this doesn't have to be at the exclusion of all others. High GI foods such as potatoes and wholemeal bread make a valuable nutritional contribution to your diet, and when eaten with protein foods or low GI carbs the overall GI value of the meal will be about medium.

What's the GI of eggs and cheese?

There is no point wondering about the GI of eggs and cheese—these foods don't have one. It is not scientifically possible to measure a GI value for foods that contain negligible carbohydrate.

Does a food's GI value make it good or bad for you?

When choosing foods, the GI is not intended to be used on its own. A food's GI value doesn't make it good or bad for you. The nutritional benefits of different foods are many and varied. We suggest you base your food choices on the overall nutritional content, along with the amount of saturated fat, salt, fiber and, of course, the GI value.

Should I use GI or GL? What's the difference and does it really matter?

We are often asked this question. Your blood glucose rises and falls when you eat a food or meal containing carbohydrate. How high it rises and how long it remains high depends on the quality of the carbohydrate (its GI) as well as the *quantity* of carbohydrate in your meal. Researchers at Harvard University came up with a term that combines these two factors—glycemic load (GL). So which one—GI or GL —should you use?

Our advice is to stick with the GI rather than GL, the reason being that following the low GL route may lead you straight to a low carb diet that doesn't incorporate the benefits of low GI foods. If you choose low GI carbs, you'll find that you are automatically reducing the GL of your diet and at the same time you'll feel more satisfied and have a diet that's healthier in many other respects. A low carb diet will not necessarily have these attributes.

We also emphasize that there is no need to get overly technical about this. Think of the GI as a tool allowing you to choose one food over another in the same food group—the best bread to choose, the best cereal to choose, etc—and don't get bogged down with figures. A low GI diet is about eating a wide variety of healthy foods that fuel our bodies best—these are the less processed and wholesome foods that will provide carbs in a slow-release form.

Does low carb automatically mean low GI?

Not at all. Here's why. Low carb is just about quantity; it simply means that a food or meal does not contain much carbohydrate at all. It says nothing about the quality of the carbs in the food or meal on your plate. You will be eating more saturated fat and missing out on the benefits of slow carbs.

Low GI, on the other hand, is all about quality. Whether you are a moderate or high carb eater, low GI carbs (whole grain breads, legumes, many fruits and vegetables) will have significant health benefits—promoting weight control, reducing your blood and insulin levels throughout the day, and increasing your sense of feeling full and satisfied after eating. We suggest that you make the most of quality carbs and reap the added health benefits such as:

- vitamin E from whole grain cereals
- vitamin C, beta-carotene and potassium from fruits and vegetables
- vitamin B_6 from bananas and whole grain cereals
- pantothenic acid, zinc, iron and magnesium from whole grains and legumes
- antioxidants and phytochemicals from all plant foods
- fiber, which comes from all of the above and doesn't come from any animal food.

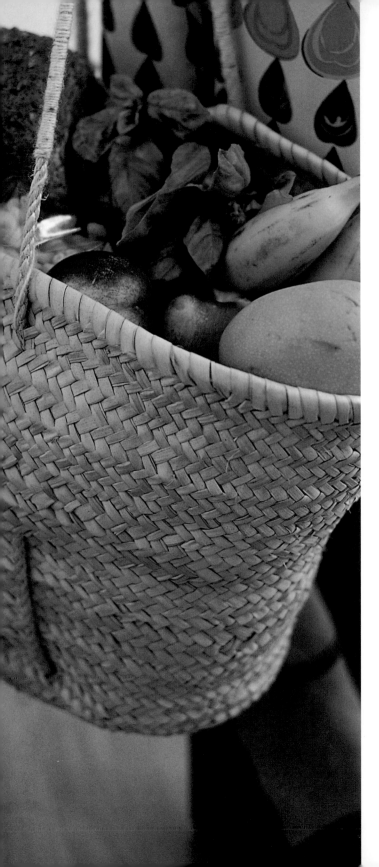

Making the switch to low GI eating

It's easy. It has science on its side. There are no strict rules or daily diet plans to follow. It's essentially about making simple modifications to your usual eating habits—such as swapping one bread for another one, or one breakfast cereal for another; for example, eating muesli for breakfast instead of wheat flakes.

Although the glycemic index itself has a scientific basis, you don't need to count numbers or do any sort of mental arithmetic to make sure you are eating a healthy low GI diet. With low GI eating, you'll find that you are enjoying foods from all the food groups and reaping the benefits of more than 40 nutrients. You'll also be taking in the protective antioxidants and phytochemicals your body needs each day for long-term health and well-being.

"This for that" table

Simply replacing high GI foods with low GI alternatives will give your overall diet a low GI and deliver the benefits of low GI eating. The following table demonstrates how you can put those low GI carbs to work in your day by cutting back consumption of high GI foods and replacing them with alternatives that are just as tasty—if not more so.

This for that

If you are currently eating this (high GI) food...	...choose this (low GI) alternative instead
Biscuits	A slice of whole grain bread or toast with jam, fruit spread or a nut spread
Breads such as soft white or wholemeal; smooth-textured breads, rolls, scones	Dense breads with whole grains, whole grain and stone-ground flour, sourdough; look for low GI labelling
Breakfast cereals—most commercial, processed cereals including corn flakes, rice crispies and cereal "biscuits"	Traditional rolled oats, muesli and the commercial low GI brands; look for low GI labelling
Cakes and pastries	Raisin toast and fruit buns, particularly the whole grain varieties; yogurts and low fat mousses also make great snacks or desserts
Chips and other packaged snacks, such as pretzels	Fresh fruit, dried fruit and nuts
Crackers	Crisp vegetable strips such as carrot, pepper and celery
Doughnuts and croissants	Try a skim milk cappuccino or smoothie instead
French fries	Leave them out! Have salad or extra vegetables instead. Corn on the cob or bean salad are better take-out options to accompany your meals
Lollipops	Chocolate is lower GI but high in fat. Healthier options are raisins, dried apricots and other dried fruits
Muesli bars	Try a nut bar or a dried fruit and nut mix
Potatoes	Prepare smaller amounts of potato. Canned new potatoes are an easy and lower GI option, or a potato salad made with cold potatoes and a vinaigrette dressing. You can also try sweet potato, yam or taro—or just replace with other low carb vegetables such as carrot, pumpkin and greens. If you can't do without your mashed potato, try replacing half the potato with cannellini beans—a white starchy bean with a low GI
Rice, especially large serves of it in dishes such as risotto, nasi goreng and fried rice	Try basmati rice, Japanese koshikari rice, pearl barley, cracked wheat (bulgur), quinoa, pasta or noodles
Soft drinks and fruit juice drinks	Try replacing these with plain mineral or soda water with a squeeze of lemon or lime juice. Fruit juice has a lower GI (but it is not a lower calorie option). If you choose juice, dilute with water or mineral or soda water. Plain water is best.
Sugar	Moderate the quantity. Consider pure floral honey, apple juice, fructose, grape nectar and agave nectar as alternatives. Adding extra fruit or dried fruit to cakes and muffins can reduce the amount of sugar needed and increase their nutritional value.

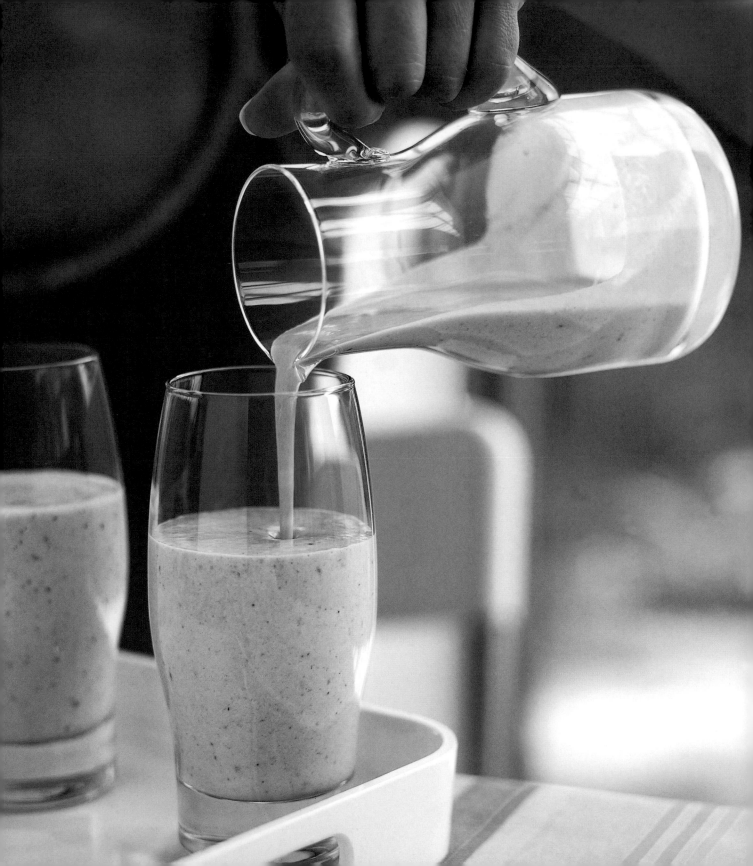

the healthy veggie

Vegetarian eating isn't just about cutting out meat and surviving on lentils or steamed vegetables. A well-balanced vegetarian or vegan diet means choosing a wide variety of foods from all the food groups to delight the taste buds and nourish the body.

In this chapter we show you how to combine the basics of healthy vegetarian and vegan eating with the benefits of low GI carbs, along with some meal ideas to help you make the switch to low GI eating. There's also a week of menus for vegetarian and vegan adults, teenagers and children, putting it all together for everybody, every day.

The healthy veggie guidelines

Every day:

- Eat seven or more servings of fruit and vegetables

  (five servings of vegetables and two servings of fruit).

- Make the most of whole grain breads and cereals with a low GI.

- Include a variety of plant proteins.

- Make sure you eat a handful of nuts regularly.

- Choose low fat dairy products or calcium-enriched alternatives.

- Opt for monounsaturated and omega-3 polyunsaturated fats

  such as olive and canola oil, and those found in nuts, seeds

  and avocado.

Eat seven or more servings of vegetables and fruit

Fruit and vegetables are recommended as the basis of all healthy diets. They are low-calorie, fiber-rich foods, containing an abundance of vitamins, minerals, antioxidants and phytochemicals. There is no disputing that a diet based on fruit and vegetables is good for our health and can help to protect us against diseases such as cancer and cardiovascular disease.

The GI is most relevant for those who eat large quantities of starchy, high-carbohydrate vegetables. Of these, the potato—the staple of Western diets—has the highest GI, whereas taro and yam have low GI values. This means that if you are a big potato eater, you should try to replace some potato for these lower GI vegetables. Apart from starchy vegetables such as potato, sweet potato, corn, taro and yam, most vegetables have very little carbohydrate and therefore do not have a GI value, or their GI can't be measured. Pumpkin and parsnips have a high GI value but there is little carbohydrate in a normal-sized serving.

As for green and salad vegetables, eat them freely. Aim to eat at least five servings each day (one serving is half a cup of cooked vegetables or one cup of salad vegetables).

Remember, variety is the key. Beans, carrots and peas are delicious, but there's a wonderful range of vegetables out there in your green-grocer, supermarket or fresh-produce store. Buy something different each time you shop—baby spinach, baby bok choy, broccoli or broccolini, cauliflower, cabbage, Brussels sprouts, pepper, fennel, tomato, cucumber, arugula, asparagus, zucchini, snow peas and eggplant. Aim to make your plate as colorful as possible. Check out what's in season right now.

Most fruits have a low GI thanks to the presence of the low GI sugar fructose, soluble and insoluble fibers and acids (which may slow down stomach-emptying). The lowest GI fruits are those grown in temperate climates—apples, pears, all citrus fruits and stone fruits. Generally, the more acidic a fruit, the lower the GI. Tropical fruits, such as pineapple, paw paw (papaya) and watermelon tend to have intermediate GI values, but are excellent sources of antioxidants, and in average servings their glycemic load is low. Aim for at least two serves of fruit a day—one serve is a medium piece such as an apple or banana or 2–3 small pieces such as plums.

Here are some ideas to help you enjoy your seven servings a day.

Breakfast
- Include fruit (fresh, canned in natural juice or dried) with your breakfast cereal.
- Try a fresh fruit smoothie for a quick but satisfying breakfast meal.
- For a more substantial breakfast, add some vegetables on your toast—try asparagus, mushrooms, tomato and onion, or sliced tomato and avocado.
- Mushrooms, asparagus and tomato are also good additions to omelets.

Lunch

- Add plenty of salad vegetables on your sandwich—try tomato, lettuce, cucumber, sprouts, beet, grated carrot and pepper.
- For toasted sandwiches, go for tomato, pepper, mushroom, sweet potato, olives, zucchini and eggplant.
- Use avocado as a spread on your sandwich instead of butter or margarine.
- Salads are a great way to fill up at lunchtime, and the possibilities are endless. Don't stick with lettuce, tomato and cucumber—try adding snow peas, red or green pepper, corn, green beans, steamed broccoli, asparagus, roasted sweet potato and eggplant, sun-dried tomatoes and a few cubes of avocado or some olives.

- In colder weather, soups are a great way to get more vegetables into your diet—try pumpkin, sweet potato, lentil, split pea, minestrone or tomato.

Dinner

- Include vegetables or salads with all main meals—serve them steamed, seasoned with fresh or dried herbs, or with a dressing made from olive oil, lemon juice, balsamic vinegar and garlic.
- Always have some frozen vegetables handy for when you haven't had time to shop for fresh varieties.

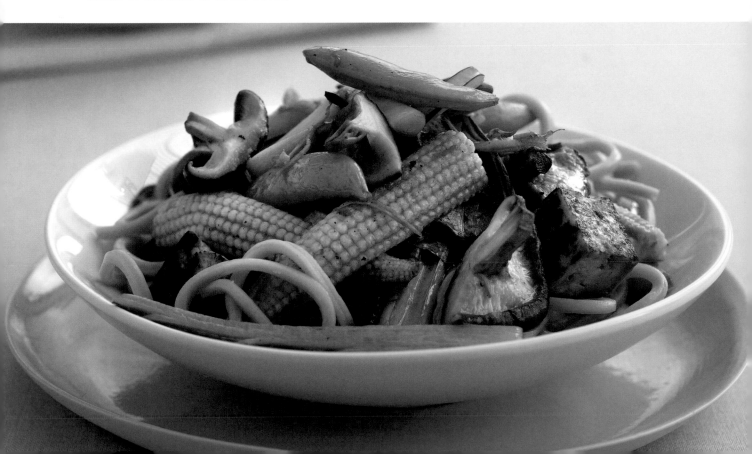

Snacks and desserts

- Fruit and grated vegetables such as carrot and zucchini can be added to cakes and muffins.
- Choose fruit for snacks—fruit is widely available, inexpensive and easy to eat, without the added fat and sugar found in many other snack foods.
- Enjoy raw vegetables such as celery, carrot, cucumber, red or green pepper, broccoli or cauliflower florets as a snack served with a hummus or salsa.
- Make fruit the basis of your desserts— try baked apples, fruit crumbles, filo with fruit, and canned fruit with low fat custard, yogurt or ice cream.

What about potatoes?

Boiled, mashed, baked or fried, everybody loves potatoes. However, we now know that the GI value of potatoes can vary significantly, depending on the variety and cooking method (the range is GI 56 to 89). Pre-cooking and reheating potatoes, or consuming cold cooked potatoes (such as potato salad with vinaigrette dressing), reduces the glycemic response. The highest GI values are found in potatoes that have been freshly cooked, and in instant mashed potatoes.

In our testing so far in Australia, the only potatoes to make the moderate GI range are tiny, new canned ones (GI 65). The lower GI of these potatoes may be due to differences in the structure of the starch.

There's no need to say no to potatoes altogether just because they may have a high GI. They are fat free (when you don't fry them), nutrient rich and filling. Not every food you eat has to have a low GI. So enjoy them, but in moderation. Try steaming small new potatoes (with their skin on for added nutrients), or bake a potato and add a tasty topping based on beans, chickpeas or corn kernels. Add variety to meals and try replacing potatoes with corn, sweet potato or yams, or serve up pasta, noodles, basmati rice or legumes.

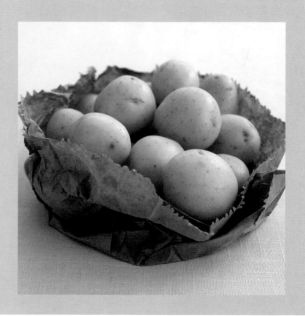

Choose whole grain breads and cereals with a low GI

Cereal grains including rice, wheat, oats, barley, rye, and products made from them (including bread, pasta, breakfast cereals and flours), are the most concentrated sources of carbohydrate we eat, and so have a major impact on the GI of our diet.

Whole grain breads and cereals have many health benefits. Most have a lower GI than refined cereal grains, and more fiber, vitamins, minerals and phytochemicals. We know too that consuming more cereal fiber and whole grains is associated with a reduced incidence of type 2 diabetes, cancer and heart disease.

What about gluten?

People with celiac disease have a permanent intolerance of gluten, a type of protein in wheat, rye, barley, millet, triticale and oats. Even eating tiny amounts can cause a problem. There are a number of gluten-free products on the market, but with their refined corn or rice starch content, many have medium or high GI values. Some have been tested for their GI—but not all. We suggest you keep foods such as rice, corn or brown rice pasta for a treat. If you are on a gluten-free diet and need to reduce the overall GI of your diet, opt for basmati rice or noodles made from rice or mung beans, combined with chickpeas and legumes.

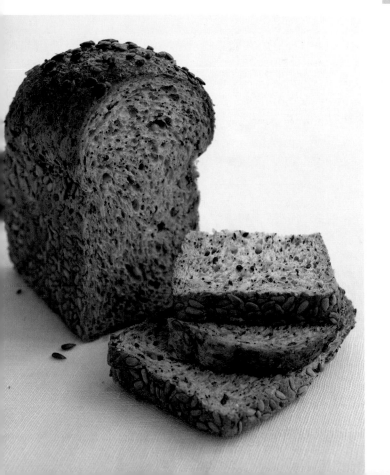

Unfortunately, our Western diet tends to be based on highly processed grains and flours, which are quickly digested and result in a much greater rise in blood glucose and insulin levels than is desirable. Since high insulin levels are something you want to avoid, replacing processed grains and cereals for those with a lower GI is a very important part of making the change to a healthy, vegetarian, low GI diet. Lower GI choices include oats, whole grain and sourdough breads, bulgur, barley, quinoa, most types of pasta and noodles, and longer-grain varieties of rice such as basmati.

Here are some ideas to help you eat more whole grain cereals and breads with a low GI.

Breakfast

- Oatmeal is one of the best breakfast choices around—it is inexpensive, has no added fats or sugars and is really satisfying, particularly on a cold morning. Add some stewed apple, a few raisins and a sprinkle of cinnamon for sweetness, and top with low fat milk or soy milk. Remember to choose whole oats rather than the instant varieties, which have a much higher GI due to all that processing.
- In warmer weather choose cereals based on wheat bran, psyllium and oats, such as natural muesli and All-Bran™.
- For those who prefer toast, choose grainy bread, pumpernickel or sourdough.

Lunch

- For sandwiches, go for grainy breads made with barley, rye, flaxseed, triticale, sunflower seed, oats, soy and cracked wheat. You could also try sourdough or pumpernickel breads.
- Barley can be added to soups to make a satisfying winter lunch.
- Falafel (made from chickpeas) and tabbouli (made from cracked wheat) make a tasty lunch combined with hummus inside wholemeal pita bread.
- Use whole grain English muffins to make mini pizzas topped with tomato, peppers, mushrooms, avocado, a few olives and a sprinkle of grated cheese or thinly sliced tofu.
- Lunching out? Try a small pasta with a tomato-based sauce, or an Asian noodle soup.

Dinner

- Choose Asian noodles, rice or egg noodles in place of rice.
- If you do want rice, try a medium GI rice such as basmati.
- Barley can be added to soups and casseroles or used in place of rice—it has a nutty, chewy texture.
- Use wholemeal or white pita breads to make an instant pizza base—top with tomato paste, mushrooms, pepper, olives and a sprinkle of parmesan cheese.

Snacks and desserts

- Whole grain raisin toast with ricotta makes a satisfying snack for those with a sweet tooth.
- Baked wholemeal or white pita bread served with salsa or hummus is a healthy alternative to chips.
- Try whole grain crispbreads topped with ricotta, avocado or hummus, and sliced tomato.
- For dessert you could try a fruit crumble with oat topping, creamed rice made with medium GI rice, or bread and butter pudding.

Rice

Rice can have a very high GI value, or a low one, depending on the variety and its amylose content. Amylose is a kind of starch that resists gelatinization. Although rice is a whole grain food, when you cook it, the millions of microscopic cracks in the grains let water penetrate right to the middle of the grain, allowing the starch granules to swell and become fully 'gelatinized', thus very easy to digest.

So, if you are a big rice eater, opt for a low GI variety with a higher amylose content, such as basmati. High-amylose rices stay firm and separate when cooked, and they combine well with Indian, Thai and Vietnamese cuisines.

Brown rice is an extremely nutritious form of rice and contains several B vitamins, minerals, dietary fibre and protein. Chewier than regular white rice, it tends to take about twice as long to cook. Most varieties that have been tested to date have a high or medium GI, so try to combine brown rice with low GI foods in your meal. Arborio risotto rice releases its starch during cooking and has a medium GI. Wild rice (GI 57) is not actually rice at all, but a type of grass seed.

As with pasta and noodles, it's all too easy to overeat rice, so keep portions moderate. Even when you choose a low GI rice, eating too much can have a marked effect on your blood glucose. A cup of cooked rice combined with plenty of mixed vegetables can turn into three cups of a rice-based meal that suits any adult's daily diet.

Why 'gelatinization' means high GI

The starch in raw carb-rich foods such as rice grains is stored in hard, compact granules that make the food difficult to digest unless you cook it. This is why eating raw potatoes can give you a stomachache. During cooking, water and heat expand starch granules to different degrees; some actually burst and free the molecules. This happens when you make gravy by heating flour and water until the starch granules burst and the gravy thickens. If most of the starch granules have swollen during cooking, we say that the starch is fully gelatinized. It is now also easy to digest, which is why the food will have a high GI.

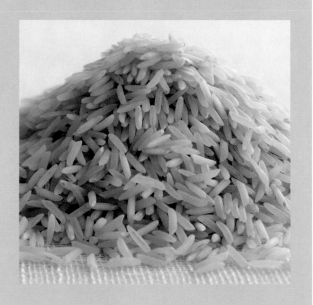

Include a variety of sources of protein in your diet

How's this for variety—legumes, tofu, eggs, seitan, Quorn™, TVP, tempeh and vegetarian burgers and sausages? For meat eaters, the GI of protein sources such as meat, fish, chicken and eggs is not relevant because these foods don't contain carbohydrate. For the vegetarian, however, most of your protein foods are also sources of carbohydrate, and all of them, as far as we've measured, are low GI.

Legumes are the dried seeds found inside the mature pods of leguminous plants (e.g. beans, peas and lentils). Nutritionally, they are quite different from fresh, young green beans and peas, which don't have as much protein or fiber because their water content is high. They reign supreme as low GI foods, and as a vegetarian you should eat them in some form most days.

Legumes are low in fat and high in fiber—both soluble and insoluble—and are packed with nutrients, providing a valuable source of protein, carbohydrate, B vitamins, folate and minerals. Sprouted dried beans—such as mung beans, soy beans, chickpeas and lentils—are excellent sources of vitamin C and are great eaten raw in a salad or stir-fried.

You can buy legumes dried or canned. Canned legumes are ready to use (they only need heating through), while dried legumes need a little more preparation—most need to be soaked before cooking—but are worth the effort and can be frozen in small batches so they are ready to use at any time. Soaked or cooked beans can be kept in an airtight container for several days in the fridge.

All legumes, apart from broad beans, have a low GI, including dried and canned varieties, although the canned varieties tend to be a little higher than those you cook yourself.

Thanks to a tendency to cause intestinal gas, legumes have generally had a bad name. But not all legumes will cause gas, and not everyone has the problem. Cooking legumes thoroughly in fresh water (not in the water you soaked them in) and rinsing the canned varieties helps, as does eating them regularly—it can improve your tolerance.

Tofu (*soybean curd*) is an easy way of using soy. It has a mild flavor itself but absorbs the flavors of other foods, making it delicious when it has been marinated in soy sauce, ginger and garlic and tossed into a stir-fry. Tofu contains very little carbohydrate so doesn't have a GI value.

Eggs are a great source of several essential vitamins and minerals, including vitamins A, D and E and the B-group vitamins, in addition to iron, phosphorus and zinc. Their cholesterol content is only a concern if you have high cholesterol levels and/or your diet is high in saturated fat.

To enhance your intake of omega-3 fats we suggest that you eat omega-3 enriched eggs (if you can find them in your supermarket). These enriched eggs are produced by feeding the hens a diet that is naturally rich in omega-3s (including canola and flaxseeds).

Quorn™ (see page 6) is low in saturated fat and is a good source of protein, fiber, iron and zinc. It can be used in cooking, or you will find it in ready-made meals such as casseroles, pies and curries.

Seitan comes from wheat gluten and is high in protein and low in fat. When cooked, it can taste so like "meat" that it is sometimes called "wheat meat".

Tempeh is made from fermented cooked soybeans. An excellent source of protein, it also contains dietary fiber and phytochemicals. Try it sliced on sandwiches or in salads, or use it in stir-fries and curries.

TVP (*textured vegetable protein*) is made from soy flour, which is processed and dried to give a product with a sponge-like texture. It is prepared by adding water or stock and can then be used as a meat substitute in a variety of dishes. It is also often incorporated into vegetarian burgers, sausages and canned foods.

There are a variety of vegetarian burgers, patties, sausages and schnitzels available which are made from legumes or soy products. These provide a convenient source of protein and other vitamins and minerals for those who are time-pressed. Keep these as occasional convenience foods, as most tend to be high in salt and some can also be quite high in fat.

Breakfast
- Scrambled egg on toast—team with grilled tomato, sautéed mushrooms or steamed asparagus for a satisfying start to the day.
- Or try scrambling silken tofu in place of eggs—add some fresh or dried herbs and chopped tomato, and sauté in a little olive oil.
- Try an omelet filled with pepper and mushrooms.

Lunch
- Eggs make great sandwich fillings—try sliced boiled egg with salad, or curried egg and lettuce.
- A vegetable frittata can be served hot or cold with salad.
- Try a wrap with slices of tempeh or marinated tofu and salad.
- A veggie burger with salad on a whole grain roll makes a quick and easy lunch option for work or school.
- Lentil, split pea or minestrone soup all make a satisfying winter lunch.
- Add a can of three-bean mix or some chickpeas to create a salad that really fills you up.
- A vegetarian sausage on a grainy roll with beans and grated cheese will be a favorite with the kids.

Dinner

- Serve red kidney beans with tacos, burritos, pasta or rice.
- Chickpeas have a nutty flavor and go well in curries and stir-fries.
- Make some dahl (lentils cooked with spices) to accompany your next curry.
- Green soybeans (*edamame*) make a tasty addition to a stir-fry—they can be bought frozen in most Asian grocery stores.
- Add cannellini, borlotti or black-eyed beans to stews and casseroles.
- Firm tofu can be cubed, marinated and added to stir-fries or threaded onto skewers with vegetables to make kebabs for the barbecue or grill.
- Quorn™, seitan and tempeh can be used in stir-fries, casseroles and curries.

- Use TVP to make traditional ground meat-based dishes including lasagna, spaghetti bolognaise, cottage pie and chili con carne.
- Vegetarian sausages and marinated tofu kebabs are great for the barbecue.

Snacks and desserts

- Silken tofu can be used in place of cream cheese to make desserts such as cheesecake.
- Roasted chickpeas or soybeans make a tasty and satisfying snack.
- For a healthy dip, go for hummus or bean purée spread and serve with carrot and celery sticks.

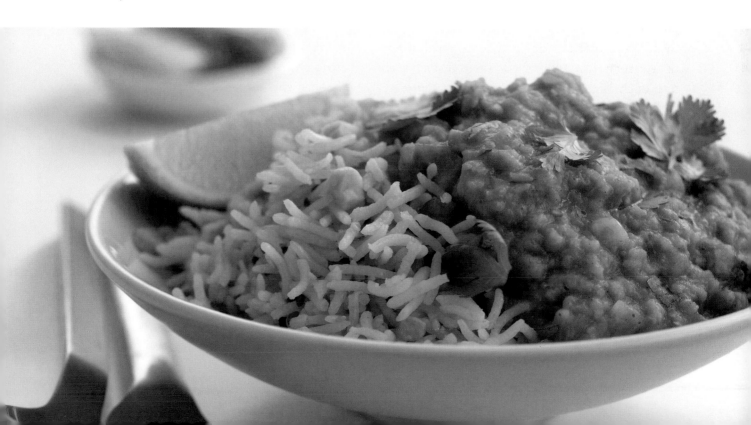

Include nuts and seeds regularly in your diet

Nuts are a food that most people enjoy but few people eat regularly, particularly if they are watching their weight. The good news is that a number of studies have now shown a relationship between regular nut consumption and a reduced risk of both heart disease and type 2 diabetes.

For vegetarians, nuts are an excellent source of protein, iron and zinc, while almonds are also a good source of calcium. They're generally not major sources of carbohydrate, although peanuts and cashews contain more carbohydrate than other nuts and have very low GI values.

Eaten in small amounts, nuts have also been shown to assist with weight control, as they are satisfying and therefore stop you snacking on other foods. Nuts are a healthy choice because they contain:

- very little saturated fat (the fats are predominantly monounsaturated or polyunsaturated)
- dietary fiber
- vitamin E, an antioxidant believed to help prevent heart disease
- folate, copper and magnesium, nutrients also thought to protect against heart disease.

Walnuts and pecans also contain some omega-3 fats, while flaxseeds are very rich in omega-3s, lignans and plant estrogens. When freshly ground, flaxseeds have a subtle nutty flavor and make a great addition to breads, muffins, biscuits and cereals.

Remember to choose the unsalted variety—salted nuts are usually roasted in saturated fat. And stick to a small handful a day if you are watching your weight. Some easy ways to eat more nuts include:

Breakfast

- Sprinkle a mixture of nuts and seeds over your cereal, or add to your muesli mix.
- Use a spread such as peanut, almond or cashew butter on your toast in place of butter or margarine.
- Add some chopped brazil nuts and pistachios to a fruit salad.
- Try grated pear and low fat natural yogurt sprinkled with sunflower and pumpkin seeds.

Lunch

- Add walnuts or pine nuts to your salad.
- Tahini (sesame seed paste) can be used as a spread on sandwiches or in salads in place of mayonnaise.

Dinner

- Add nuts and seeds to your favorite meals— try peanuts or sesame seeds in a stir-fry, cashews or crushed macadamias with a curry.
- Pesto (ground pine nuts, basil, parmesan, garlic and olive oil) makes a good pasta sauce.
- Tahini can be used as an alternative to sour cream on potatoes, or drizzled over roasted vegetables.

Snacks and desserts

- Enjoy nuts as a snack. Although high in fat, nuts make a healthy substitute for less nutritious high fat snacks such as potato chips, chocolate and biscuits. Just be careful not to eat too many—limit yourself to one handful (about 30 g/1 oz) a day.
- Whole grain crackers or toast with nut spread make a satisfying snack.
- Nuts and seeds can be added to baked foods—try walnuts, hazelnuts and almond meal in cakes and muffins, and sunflower seeds, sesame seeds and flaxseeds in bread.
- Roast sesame seeds, sunflower seeds and pumpkin seeds and toss in tahini for a wholesome snack.
- Top desserts with a sprinkle of chopped nuts such as macadamias and hazelnuts.

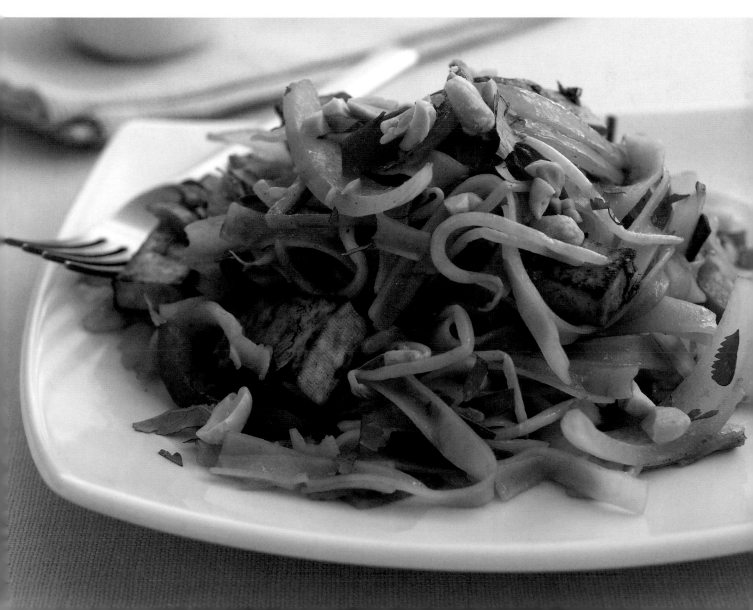

Eat low fat dairy foods and calcium-enriched alternatives

Scientists have known for years that a diet high in saturated fat raises cholesterol levels and increases heart disease risk. More recently, research has also implicated these fats in both insulin resistance and obesity—we burn saturated fat poorly compared with other fats, so it tends to be stored as body fat more readily. In contrast, our bodies are more likely to use omega-3 polyunsaturated fatty acids (PUFAs) and monounsaturated fatty acids (MUFAs) for energy rather than storage.

Reducing your intake of saturated fat doesn't mean that you need to avoid dairy products. So as long as you choose low fat dairy products you can still include these foods in moderation as part of a healthy diet. Dairy products, including milk, yogurt and cheese, are among the richest sources of calcium in our diet. They also provide protein, and a number of important vitamins and minerals including vitamin B_{12}, phosphorus, magnesium and zinc.

As an alternative to dairy foods you could choose calcium-fortified soy products, such as soy milk and soy yogurt. As a vegetarian, it is also good to try to choose one with added vitamin B_{12}. Soy products contain mostly polyunsaturated fat, and the protein in soy products can help to lower cholesterol levels. Soy products are also a source of omega-3 fatty acids and phytoestrogens. When purchasing soy products, check labels for total fat content of no more than 3–5 percent.

You can include low fat dairy and soy products in your diet in the following ways:

Breakfast
- Fruit smoothies make a great breakfast when you are on the go.
- Low fat yogurt (plain or flavored) is a tasty accompaniment to muesli.
- Make oatmeal with low fat milk and add a dollop of yogurt to serve.
- Labneh (spreadable yogurt) makes a tasty topping for grainy toast.

Lunch
- Sandwiches or rolls can be filled with avocado, tomato and cheese, or ricotta, sun-dried tomato and arugula.
- Dress up your salad with some cubes of low fat feta cheese or baked ricotta.

Protection from plants

Phytoestrogens are natural plant chemicals found in foods such as fruit, vegetables, nuts and soy foods. Research shows that people who consume high levels of phytoestrogens enjoy better health and live longer. Phytoestrogens can help to reduce the symptoms of menopause and can lower cholesterol levels and protect against cancer. You can increase your intake of phytoestrogens by eating legumes, tofu and nuts regularly, switching from dairy to soy milk and eating breads and cereals containing soy and flaxseed.

Dinner

- Low fat yogurt and ricotta mixed with chives makes a low fat alternative to sour cream on vegetables or Mexican food.
- Light evaporated milk thickened with cornstarch makes a great white sauce for pastas and vegetable mornays. With 1–2 spoonfuls of dried coconut, it can be used as a low fat alternative to coconut milk.
- Soy milk can also be used in place of milk for making white sauces and creamy soups.
- Ricotta and spinach lasagna or manicotti will be a favorite with vegetarians and non-vegetarians alike.
- Sprinkle low fat mozzarella or soy cheese on a roasted vegetable pizza.
- Shavings of parmesan add flavor to your favorite salad or pasta dish.

Snacks and desserts

- Fruit smoothies or low fat milkshakes make a satisfying calcium-packed snack.
- Yogurt is always a quick and easy option.
- Try a glass of low fat hot chocolate to satisfy those chocolate cravings.
- Low fat flavored milk or soy milk makes a good snack on the run.
- Ricotta can be used as a topping for crackers or spread on raisin toast.
- Add a spoonful of low fat custard, frozen yogurt or ice cream to fruit for dessert.
- Low fat ricotta can also be used in cheesecakes or as a topping for fresh fruit.

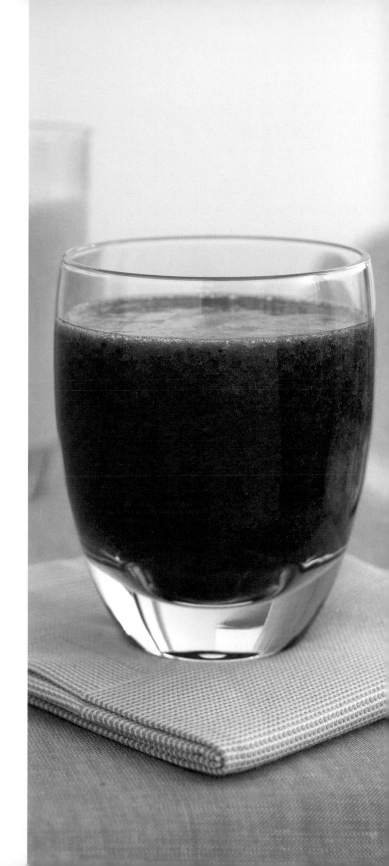

Cheese

Cheese is perfect for sandwich fillings, snacks and toppings for pasta and with gratin dishes, but it also contributes a fair amount of fat. Most cheese is around 30 percent fat, much of it saturated.

Ricotta and cottage cheese are good low fat choices—usually less than 7 percent fat content. Use them as an alternative to butter or margarine for sandwiches. It's worth trying fresh ricotta from a deli—you may find its soft, creamy texture and fresh flavor tastier than pre-packaged ricotta. When making lasagna, use creamy ricotta instead of white sauce. Flavored cottage cheese or natural cottage cheese with freshly snipped chives or basil and some black pepper make ideal low fat toppings for toast and crackers as snacks and light lunches.

Although there are a number of good reduced fat cheeses available, others can lose out in the flavor stakes for a relatively small reduction in fat. If you are a real cheese lover and are having a hard time finding a tasty low fat one, try these tips for making the most of your higher fat cheese choices:

- Consider eating a little of a strong-flavored cheese rather than a lot of something bland and tasteless.

- Shave a few strips of fresh parmesan over pasta—a vegetable peeler does the job nicely. Grating and shaving helps a little cheese go a long way.

- Enjoy full fat cheeses in small amounts occasionally. This includes regular types of cheddar, blue vein, Swiss, brie, camembert, Colby, gouda and havarti.

- Mozzarella cheese—whole milk or part skim—may contain less fat than some reduced fat cheeses. Grate and sprinkle over stuffed vegetables such as pepper or eggplant, baked potatoes and pizzas before cooking.

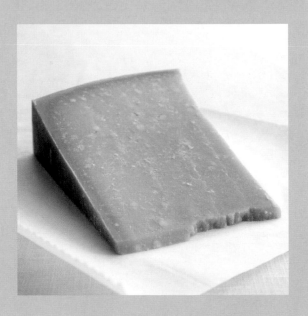

Use high omega-3 and monounsaturated oils

It is not necessary, or beneficial, to cut all fats out of your diet. In fact, some fats are essential for our health as they provide essential fatty acids and carry fat-soluble vitamins and antioxidants.

This means that it is fine to use small amounts of oil in cooking and in salad dressings, but it is important to choose the right one. If you prefer not to use oil, you could also get these "good" fats from eating nuts, seeds, avocado and olives.

When choosing oil, you want to choose types that are high in monounsaturated and omega-3 fats, such as the following:

Olive oil is high in monounsaturated fats, low in saturates and has a minimal polyunsaturated fat content, which is an advantage as it allows our bodies to make greater use of the omega-3 fats we obtain from other dietary sources, without any competition from excessive polyunsaturated omega-6 fats. Olive oil is also rich in antioxidants. It can be used in cooking or salad dressings. Olive oil margarines are also available.

Peanut oil is a mild-tasting oil that oxidizes slowly and can withstand high cooking temperatures. About 50 percent of the fat in peanut oil is monounsaturated and another 30 percent is polyunsaturated. This heart-healthy fat is good for Asian cooking, such as stir-fries.

Canola oil, besides being high in monounsaturated fat, contains significant amounts of omega-3 fats. This multipurpose cooking oil can also be used for baking. Margarine made from canola oil is also available.

Flaxseed oil is the richest plant source of omega-3s and contains very little omega-6 fats. But it is highly prone to oxidation (meaning its fats turn rancid easily), so it shouldn't be heated, and needs to be stored carefully. It is best used in salad dressings. Alternatively, flaxseeds can be freshly ground and sprinkled on cereal or added to cakes and muffins.

When choosing an oil, you also have to consider whether it is *cold-pressed*, *virgin*, *extra-virgin*, *light*, or *extra-light*. Cold-pressed oils are those that have undergone minimal processing—this means that the oil is extracted from the seed, nut or fruit by mechanical pressing only, without heat or solvents. Cold-pressed oils have a stronger flavor and color than their regular counterparts, and they're also much richer in vitamin E (a natural preservative present in oils) and other antioxidants, giving them important health benefits. For example, extra-virgin olive oil—the best quality oil made from the first cold pressing of the olives—contains 30 to 40 different antioxidants. Light and extra-light oils are light in color and flavor. The terms "light" and "extra-light" don't mean the oil is lower in fat than any other oil—all oils are 100 percent fat.

What to drink?

Water

It's calorie-free and cheap—surely two good reasons for drinking water. However, it isn't necessary to drink eight glasses a day. Food contributes at least one-third of our daily fluid requirement, so we need five to seven cups of fluid to make up the remainder. Aim to make at least two or three of these water.

Fruit juice

It is widely considered a healthy drink, but if your diet includes fruit and vegetables, fruit juice really isn't necessary. Did you know that any form of liquid energy (for example, fruit juice, soft drink) is likely to bypass satiety mechanisms in the brain? In other words, your brain ignores their energy content and you'll tend to overeat. However, if you do like to include it, one glass a day is enough, and think of it as a (low-fiber) serving of fruit.

Tea

Drinking a cup of tea often provides the opportunity to take time out and relax—there is a benefit in this. Tea has also been recognized recently as a valuable source of antioxidants, which may protect against several forms of cancer, cardiovascular disease, kidney stones, bacterial infection and dental cavities.

Herbal tea

Herbal tea is not really tea but an infusion made from the fresh or dried flowers, leaves, seeds or roots of various plants. There are many different varieties available, from chamomile to peppermint and ginger to lemon grass, some with particular health or medicinal benefits. They make a good alternative for those who like a hot drink but want to cut down on caffeine. Many herbal teas are not safe during pregnancy, so always check with your doctor or dietician before using these if you are pregnant.

Coffee

Did you know that 80 percent of the world's population consumes caffeine daily? For most people, two cups of coffee a day is fine, but if you are pregnant, caffeine sensitive or have high blood pressure it is probably best to cut down to one cup per day, or avoid it altogether. Both tea and coffee are a major source of antioxidants in the diet, simply because they are so widely and frequently consumed.

Milk or soy milk

Milk and calcium-fortified soy milks are a valuable source of nutrients for adults and children, but, being a liquid, they are easily overconsumed. Think of them as food in a liquid form. Recommended intakes vary for different ages, but for normal, healthy, non-pregnant adults, around 1–2 cups (9–16 fl oz) of low fat milk or soy milk a day is suitable.

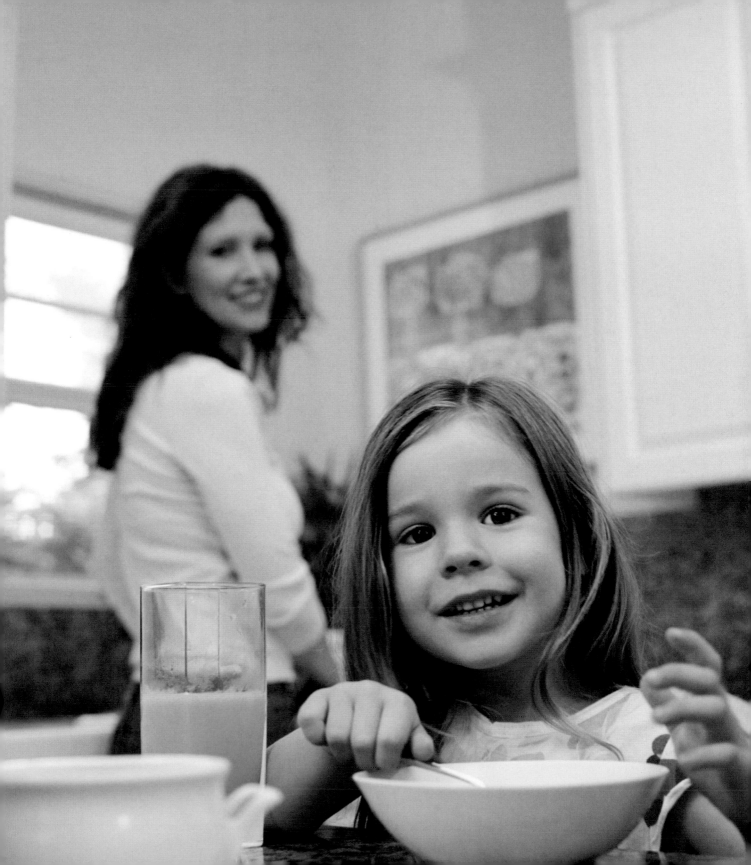

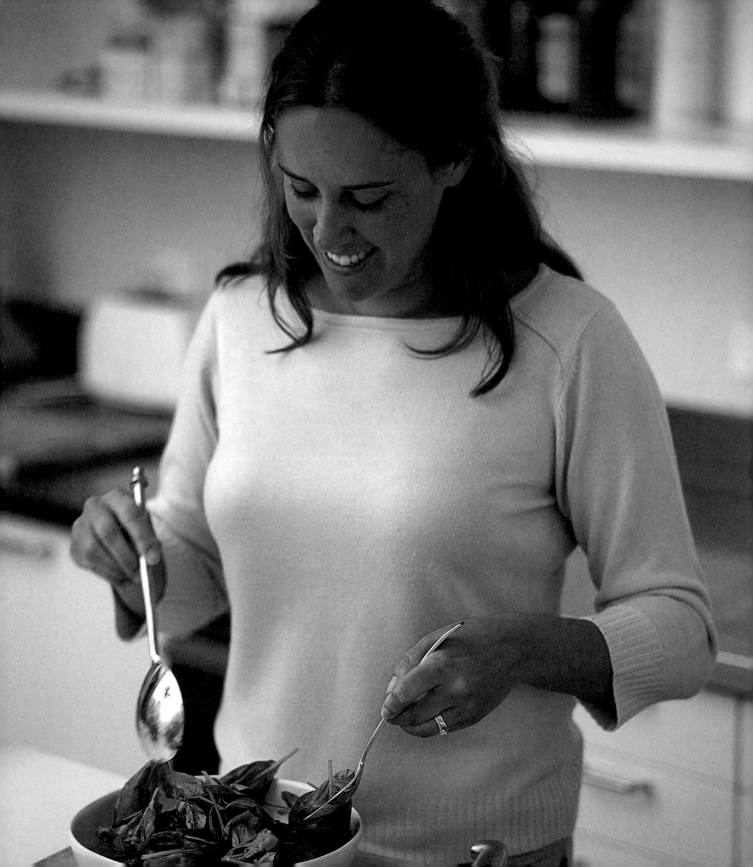

the healthy veggie menu plans

This chapter contains delicious low GI healthy veggie menus for adults, teenagers and children. We've included recipes from this book (marked with an asterisk) to inspire you, and there's an emphasis on low GI carbs, vegetarian protein, plenty of fruit and vegetables, and the good oils.

The adult menus don't include snacks, but we've suggested some for teenagers and children. The teenagers' and children's menus also reflect different taste preferences and energy needs during this vital time of growth and development. It is particularly important to monitor vitamin B_{12} intake for vegan teens and children; and if their needs aren't being met by fortified foods, see your doctor about a B_{12} supplement.

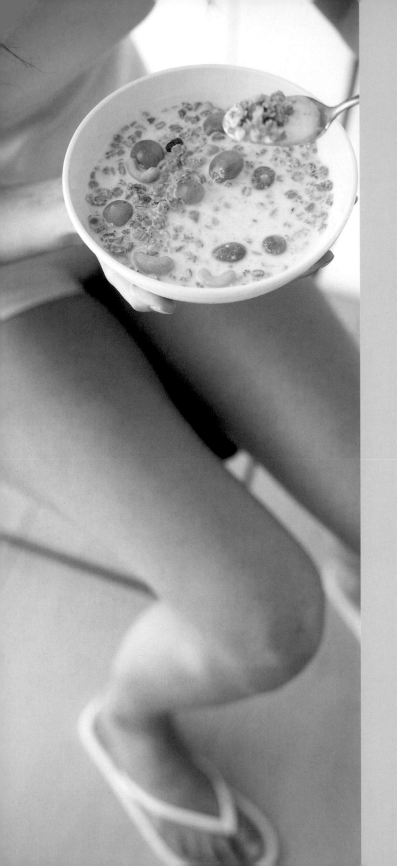

7-day menu

vegetarian adults

	breakfast	lunch	dinner
Monday	Bircher Muesli with Mango and Passionfruit*	Sourdough roll with ricotta, sundried tomato and English spinach Low fat yogurt	Chickpea and Vegetable Curry with Cumin-flavored Rice* Fresh fruit
Tuesday	Mixed-berry Breakfast Boost*	Falafel Rolls with Hummus, Tabbouleh and Spicy Tomato Sauce* Fresh fruit salad	Spiralli with Broccoli and Pesto Balsamico* Carob, Ginger and Pecan Biscotti* and a glass of milk or soy milk
Wednesday	Mixed-grain Oatmeal with Berry Compote*	Whole grain sandwich with curried egg, lettuce, snow pea sprouts and cucumber 1 apple	Bean and Corn Burritos* Apple, Cranberry and Walnut Bread* with ricotta
Thursday	Whole grain toast with avocado and tomato	Tofu, Avocado and Cucumber Sushi* Small fruit smoothie	Pumpkin, Spinach and Ricotta Manicotti* with salad Fresh fruit
Friday	Natural Nutty Muesli with Stewed Rhubarb and Ginger*	Individual Vegetable Frittata* with salad and whole grain roll	Vegetarian Pad Thai* Apple, Rhubarb and Ginger Crumble* with custard
Saturday	Asparagus and Corn Omelet*	Ricotta, Feta and Spinach Triangles* Dried fruit and nut mix	Fennel, Leek and Bean Barley Pilaf* Fresh fruit
Sunday	Rice and Cilantro Fritters*	Grilled Vegetable Skewers with Grilled Corn* Fresh fruit salad	Grilled Vegetable Pizza* with salad Fruit yogurt

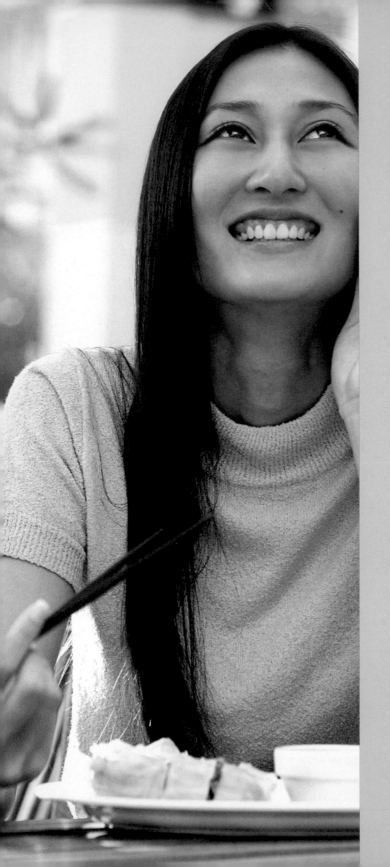

7-day menu

vegan
adults

	breakfast	lunch	dinner
Monday	Mixed-grain Oatmeal with Berry Compote*	Roasted Beet and White-bean Salad with Balsamic Dressing* and whole grain roll Fresh fruit	Vegetarian Paella* Soy hot chocolate
Tuesday	Banana and Mango Smoothie*	Vietnamese Rice-paper Rolls* Dried fruit and nut mix	Chickpea and Vegetable Curry with Cumin-flavored Rice* Baked Raisin, Date and Walnut Apple* with soy ice cream
Wednesday	Bircher Muesli with Mango and Passionfruit*	Spicy Moroccan Chickpea and Lentil Soup* with whole grain roll Fresh fruit	Vegetarian Pad Thai* Soy yogurt with berries
Thursday	Whole grain toast with avocado and tomato	Falafel Rolls with Hummus, Tabbouleh and Spicy Tomato Sauce* Soy fruit smoothie	Fennel, Leek and Bean Barley Pilaf* Fresh fruit
Friday	Natural Nutty Muesli with Stewed Rhubarb and Ginger*	Vegetarian Laksa* Fresh fruit	Three-bean Chili with Spicy Tortilla Crisps* Poached pears with soy custard
Saturday	Quinoa Oatmeal with Banana, Raisins and Pistachios* Glass of fruit juice	Lentil and Sunflower-seed Burgers* Fresh fruit	Spaghetti with Steamed Greens and White Beans* Soy hot chocolate and a handful of almonds
Sunday	Breakfast Fried Rice*	Grilled Vegetable and Tofu Salad* with whole grain roll Fresh fruit	Vegetarian Shepherd's Pie* with steamed greens Apple, Rhubarb and Ginger Crumble*

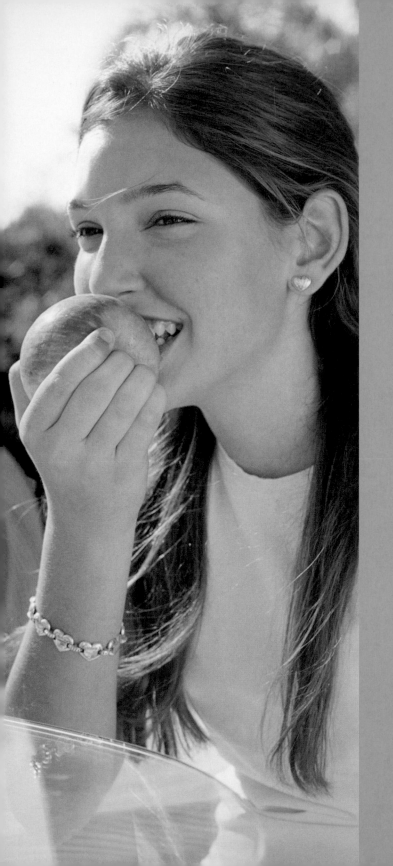

7-day menu

vegetarian teenagers

	breakfast	lunch	dinner
Monday	Mixed-grain Oatmeal with Berry Compote* and a glass of fruit juice SNACK: Dried fruit and nut mix and a banana	Whole grain egg and lettuce roll Fresh fruit SNACK: Fruit yogurt	Vegetarian Shepherd's Pie* with carrots, peas and beans Peaches and custard
Tuesday	Apple, Cranberry and Walnut Bread* and a glass of milk or soy milk SNACK: Apple and whole grain crackers with cheese	Falafel Rolls with Hummus, Tabbouleh and Spicy Tomato Sauce* Fresh fruit SNACK: Raisin toast	Grilled Vegetable Pizza* Fruit yogurt
Wednesday	Bircher Muesli with Mango and Passionfruit* SNACK: Blueberry muffin	Sourdough roll with cheese and salad Flavored milk or soy milk Fresh fruit SNACK: Toast with peanut butter	Bean and Corn Burritos* Apple, Rhubarb and Ginger Crumble* and light ice cream or soy ice cream
Thursday	Sourdough toast with peanut butter Hot chocolate with milk or soy milk SNACK: Carob, Ginger and Pecan Biscotti* and a banana	Ricotta, Feta and Spinach Triangles* with cherry tomatoes Dried fruit and nut mix SNACK: Fruit yogurt	Vegetarian Pad Thai* Fresh fruit salad
Friday	Banana and Mango Smoothie* SNACK: Whole grain crackers with cheese or peanut butter	Tofu, Avocado and Cucumber Sushi* SNACK: Raisin toast and a glass of milk or soy milk	Lentil, Mushroom and Ricotta Lasagna* Baked Raisin, Date and Walnut Apple* with custard
Saturday	Whole grain toast with baked beans SNACK: Apple and dried fruit and nut mix	Lentil and Sunflower-seed Burgers* Fresh fruit SNACK: Fruit smoothie	Three-bean Chili with Spicy Tortilla Crisps* and guacamole Fresh fruit salad
Sunday	Asparagus and Corn Omelet* SNACK: Apple	Vietnamese Rice-paper rolls* SNACK: Cheese and whole grain crackers	Lentil and Vegetable Nut Roast* Hot chocolate with milk or soy milk

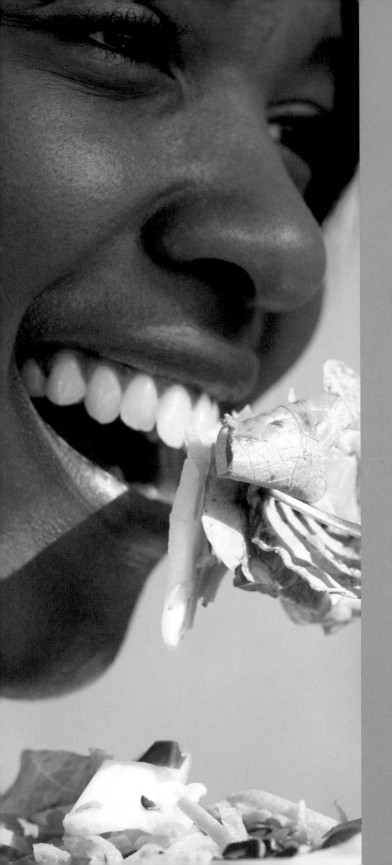

7-day menu

vegan teenagers

	breakfast	lunch	dinner
Monday	Mixed-grain Oatmeal with Berry Compote* and a glass of fruit juice SNACK: Dried fruit and nut mix and a banana	Whole grain roll with lentil burger and salad Fresh fruit SNACK: Soy yogurt	Vegetarian Shepherd's Pie* with steamed greens Peaches and soy custard
Tuesday	Whole grain toast with almond spread Glass of soy milk SNACK: Apple and a handful of nuts	Falafel Rolls with Hummus, Tabbouleh and Spicy Tomato Sauce* Fresh fruit SNACK: Raisin Toast and soy hot chocolate	Lentil and Vegetable Nut Roast* with roasted baby potatoes and steamed greens Apple, Rhubarb and Ginger Crumble* with soy ice cream
Wednesday	Bircher Muesli with Mango and Passionfruit* SNACK: Fruit salad	Sourdough roll with salad Flavored soy milk Fresh fruit SNACK: Toast with peanut butter	Red Lentil Dahl with Spiced Basmati Rice* Fruit and soy yogurt
Thursday	Sourdough toast with peanut butter Soy hot chocolate SNACK: Banana and dried fruit and nut mix	Tofu, Avocado and Cucumber Sushi* Fresh fruit SNACK: Hummus* with raw vegetables and toasted pita bread	Vegetarian Pad Thai* Fresh fruit salad
Friday	Banana and Mango Smoothie* made with soy milk SNACK: Whole grain crackers with peanut butter	Lentil and Sunflower-seed Burgers* Fresh fruit SNACK: Raisin toast and glass of soy milk	Three-bean Chili with Spicy Tortilla Crisps* Baked Raisin, Date and Walnut Apple* with soy ice cream
Saturday	Whole grain toast with baked beans SNACK: Apple and dried fruit and nut mix	Vietnamese Rice-paper Rolls* SNACK: Fruit smoothie	Spaghetti with Steamed Greens and White Beans* Fresh fruit salad
Sunday	Asian-style scrambled tofu and grilled tomato with whole grain toast SNACK: Apple	Bean and Corn Burritos* SNACK: Soy yogurt	Vegetarian Laksa* Soy hot chocolate

Note: choose soy products (milk, custard, yogurt) fortified with vitamin B$_{12}$ where possible, or provide a vitamin B$_{12}$ supplement

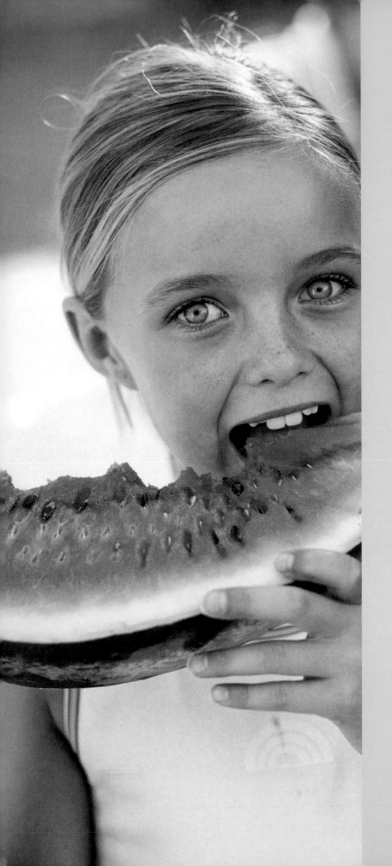

7-day menu

vegetarian children

	breakfast	lunch	dinner
Monday	Mixed-grain Oatmeal wtih Berry Compote* SNACK: Small box of raisins	Whole grain egg and lettuce roll Fruit salad SNACK: Fruit yogurt	Vegetarian Shepherd's Pie* with carrots and peas Peaches and custard
Tuesday	Sourdough toast with peanut butter and banana SNACK: Whole grain crackers with cheese	Ricotta, Feta and Spinach Triangles* Cherry tomatoes and carrot sticks SNACK: Raisin toast	Grilled Vegetable Pizza* Hot chocolate
Wednesday	Corn and Zucchini Muffins* Glass of milk or soy milk SNACK: Banana	Sourdough roll with cheese and lettuce Orange slices SNACK: Toast with peanut butter	Lentil and Vegetable Nut Roast* with green beans Fresh fruit salad
Thursday	Whole grain toast with grilled cheese and tomato SNACK: Grapes	Falafel Rolls with Hummus, Tabbouleh and Spicy Tomato Sauce* Apple SNACK: Glass of milk	Shiitake, Ginger and Tofu Hokkien Noodles* Fresh strawberries with yogurt
Friday	Banana and Mango Smoothie* SNACK: Blueberry Muffin*	Whole grain roll with peanut butter, raisins and grated carrot Kiwi fruit SNACK: Fruit yogurt	Bean and Corn Burritos* Apple crumble with ice cream
Saturday	Scrambled eggs and grilled tomato on sourdough toast SNACK: Orange	Cheese and baked bean whole grain toasted sandwich SNACK: Apple, Cranberry and Walnut Bread* and a glass of milk	Pumpkin, Spinach and Ricotta Manicotti* Banana split
Sunday	Mixed Berry Buttermilk Pancakes* SNACK: Apple and slice of cheese	Individual Vegetable Fritatta* SNACK: Chewy Fig and Apricot Granola Bars*	Vegetarian Fried Rice* Fresh fruit salad

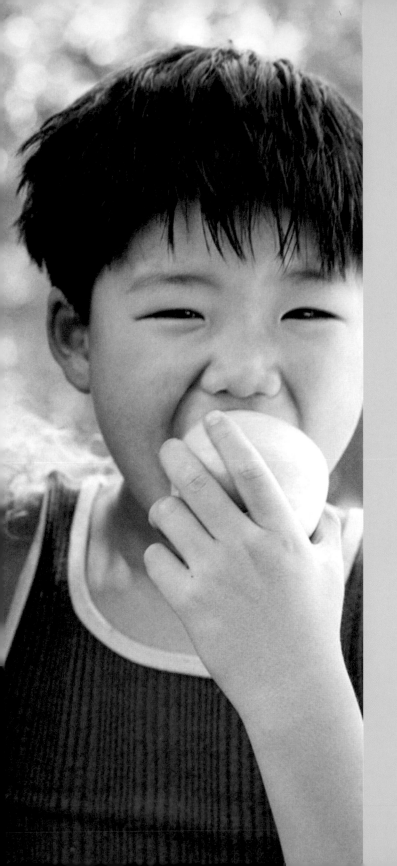

7-day menu

vegan
children

	breakfast	lunch	dinner
Monday	Mixed-grain Oatmeal with Berry Compote* SNACK: Small box of raisins	Whole grain roll with lentil burger and lettuce Fruit salad SNACK: Soy yogurt	Grilled Vegetable Skewers with Grilled Corn* and brown rice Peaches and soy custard
Tuesday	Sourdough toast with peanut butter and banana SNACK: Apple	Vietnamese Rice-paper Rolls* SNACK: Raisin toast	Vegetarian Shepherd's Pie* Soy hot chocolate
Wednesday	Whole grain cereal with soy milk and sliced banana SNACK: Handful of dried fruit	Sourdough roll with salad Orange slices SNACK: Toast with peanut butter	Vegetarian Fried Rice* Fresh fruit salad
Thursday	Whole grain toast with baked beans SNACK: Grapes	Falafel Rolls with Hummus, Tabbouleh and Spicy Tomato Sauce* Apple SNACK: Glass of soy milk with carob powder	Shiitake, Ginger and Tofu Hokkien Noodles* Fresh strawberries
Friday	Banana smoothie made with soy milk SNACK: Whole grain crackers with peanut butter	Whole grain roll with peanut butter, raisins and grated carrot Kiwi fruit SNACK: Soy yogurt	Bean and Corn Burritos* Apple crumble with soy custard
Saturday	Scrambled tofu and grilled tomato on sourdough toast SNACK: Orange	Baked bean whole grain toasted sandwich SNACK: Raisins and a glass of soy milk	Lentil and Sunflower-seed Burgers* with steamed baby potatoes and greens Banana split with soy ice cream
Sunday	Bircher Muesli with Mango and Passionfruit* and soy milk SNACK: Apple	Vegetarian pita pizzas with soy cheese SNACK: Fruit smoothie	Spaghetti with Steamed Greens and Cranberry Beans* Fresh fruit salad

Note: choose soy products (milk, custard, yogurt) fortified with vitamin B$_{12}$ where possible, or provide a vitamin B$_{12}$ supplement

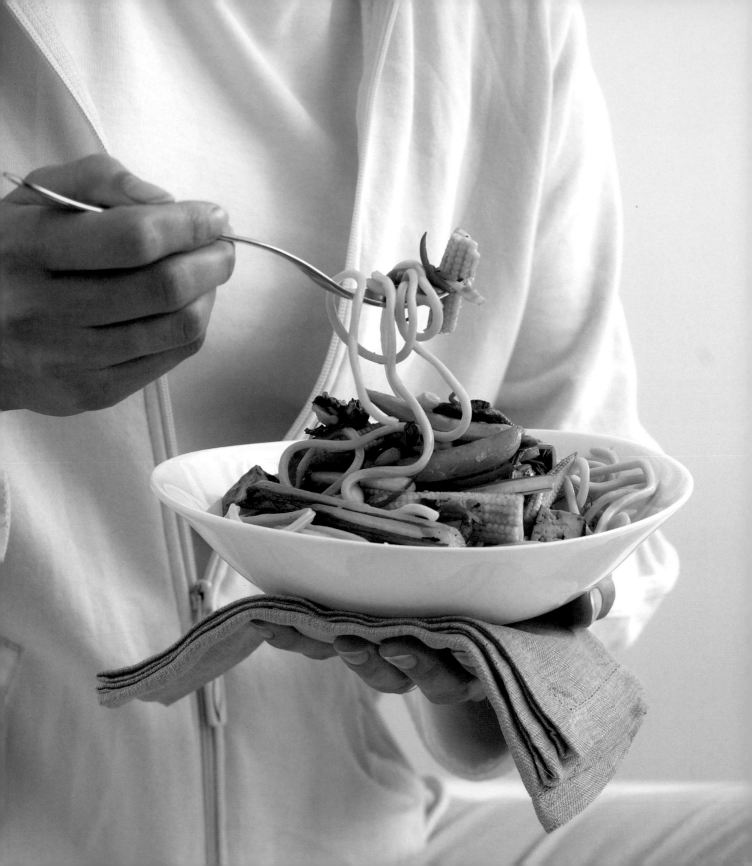

part two

recipes with a healthy balance

Cooking the low GI way

One of the aims of our books is to illustrate how to go about lowering the GI of your diet. For those who like to cook, low GI recipes are part of the picture. Even if you don't like following recipes, they can give you ideas of how to use low GI foods in flavorful and nutritious combinations.

Naturally, we aim to develop recipes that have as low a GI as possible, but there are a few popular dishes for which even we find this difficult! Typically these are baked goods made with flour, like pancakes, muffins and doughs. Because flour is a finely milled cereal product it is rapidly digested and carries a high GI. By incorporating lower GI carbs such as oat bran, whole grains, fruits, milk and juices into these recipes, we can lower the GI of these items.

Modern diets contain much more sodium (salt) than is commensurate with good health, so one of our guidelines is to limit sodium intake. We have done so in our recipes.

Each recipe is accompanied by a nutrient profile* which gives you a snapshot of its key nutritional attributes. The profile relates to a single serving, assuming you divide the recipe to make the specified number of servings. If you eat a double or triple serving of the recipe, then you would scale up the figures two or three times, respectively. The nutrient profile includes:

Energy

This is the measure of the calorie count per serving. The smaller the number, the fewer calories (or fuel) in a serving. This is a good thing if you have a tendency to gain weight. By incorporating lots of vegetables, salads, fruits and whole grains into the recipes, we've ensured that many have a low energy density. This means they are bulky and filling without providing lots of calories.

Fat

The fat content is given in grams per serving. This may be of interest if you are trying to eat a low fat diet. If the figure seems a little high to you, rest assured it is "good" fat of a poly- or monounsaturated nature. A low saturated fat intake is recommended for everyone, and all our recipes are low in saturated fat.

Protein

As a vegetarian you may be interested in the adequacy of your protein intake, so the amount of protein per serving in grams is also included. Refer to the guidelines on pages 4–7 for the recommended daily protein intake.

Carbohydrates

The amount of carbohydrates per serving in grams may be of most interest to those with diabetes. Because the GI only relates to the carbohydrate content of foods, you will find that most of our recipes have a significant carbohydrate content. It is normal and healthy for a vegetarian diet to be high in carbohydrates, but we recommend choosing predominantly low GI carbs.

*Nutrient analysis was performed using nutrient analysis software, FoodWorks ® (Xyris Software), based on Australian and New Zealand food composition data.

Fiber

It would be unusual for a vegetarian diet to contain too little fiber, but this is a common dietary problem for non-vegetarians. Because of this we have included fiber per serving in grams in the nutrient profile. The recommended daily intake is at least 30 grams.

Measurements

Recipes use large eggs with an average of 60 g (about 2 oz). All herbs used in the recipes are fresh unless otherwise stated. When we add fresh herbs to recipes we have chosen to use cup measures rather than take the less specific "handful" or "small bunch" approach. And if you opt to measure by tablespoons, you run the risk of losing count. To give you an idea, $\frac{1}{4}$ cup chopped fresh herbs would be around 5 tablespoons.

If you have a small measuring pitcher, $\frac{1}{2}$ cup chopped herbs will take you to the 4 fl oz mark on your small pitcher, and 1 cup to the 9 fl oz mark.

If you don't have a measuring cup or small pitcher, use a teacup, small coffee mug, or small plastic container like a cleaned yogurt container that holds 9 fl oz liquid.

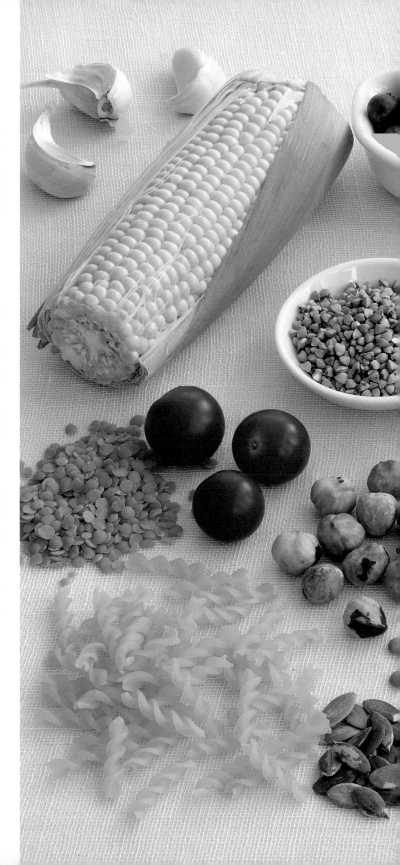

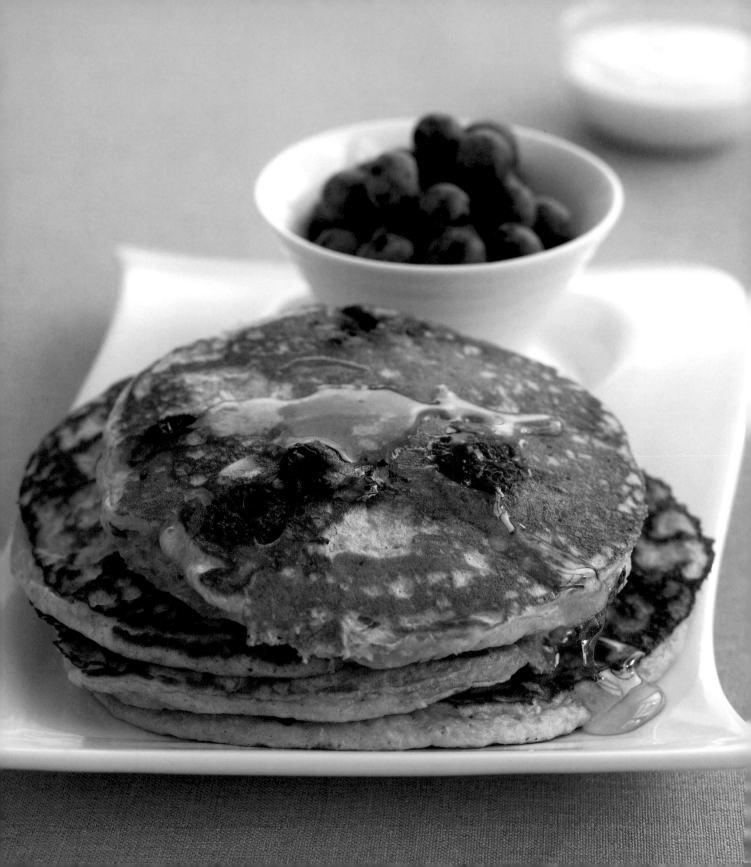

breakfasts and brunches

No doubt you know it's a good idea to eat breakfast if you want to stay healthy, but did you realize that your food choices may also be a critical factor? Firing up your engine with high GI crispy flakes or white toast provides a short-lived fuel supply that will send you in search of a fill-up within a few hours. If you want something to nourish your body, recharge your brain, speed up your metabolism and sustain you right through the morning, try our breakfast basics.

banana and mango smoothie

Serves 2 Preparation time: 10 minutes

1 large, ripe banana, chopped
1 large, ripe mango, flesh removed and chopped
1 tablespoon wheat germ
1 cup low fat milk or light soy milk, chilled
½ cup low fat natural yogurt
  or soy yogurt
2 teaspoons pure floral honey, pure maple syrup or
  rice syrup
¼ teaspoon ground cinnamon

Combine all the ingredients in a blender and blend until smooth. Pour into two tall glasses and serve.

242 Cal, 1 g fat (saturated 0 g),
3 g fiber, 13 g protein, 44 g carbohydrate

mixed-berry breakfast boost

Serves 2 Preparation time: 5 minutes

1 cup frozen mixed berries
2 scoops (4½ oz) low fat frozen yogurt or
  lemon sorbet
1½ cups freshly squeezed orange juice

Combine all the ingredients in a blender and blend until smooth. Pour into two tall glasses and serve.

159 Cal, 1 g fat (saturated 0 g),
2 g fiber, 6 g protein, 30 g carbohydrate

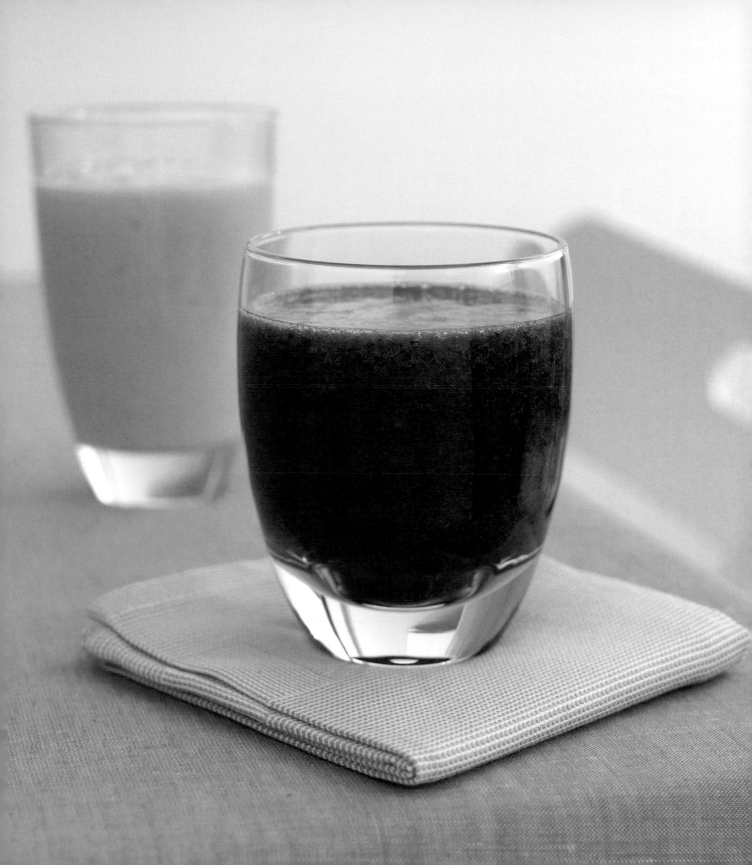

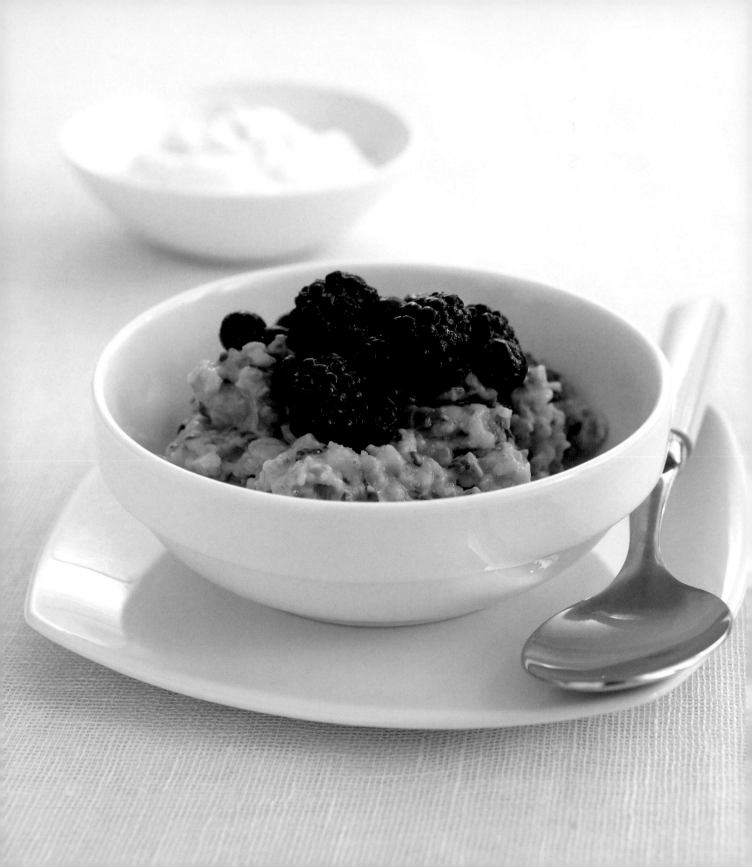

quinoa oatmeal with banana, raisins and pistachios

Serves 4   Preparation time: 10 minutes
Cooking time: 15 minutes

1 cup quinoa
2 cups low fat milk or light soy milk
1/3 cup raisins, finely chopped
1/2 teaspoon ground cinnamon
1 tablespoon pure floral honey, pure maple syrup or
  rice syrup
1 banana, sliced, to serve
1/2 cup low fat vanilla or soy yogurt,
  to serve
1/4 cup unsalted pistachios, finely chopped, to serve
low fat milk or light soy milk, extra, to serve

1. Place the quinoa in a sieve and rinse well under cold running water. Tip the quinoa into a saucepan and add the milk. Bring to a boil, then reduce the heat and simmer for 5 minutes. Add the raisins and cinnamon and simmer for 8–10 minutes, or until all of the liquid is absorbed. Stir in the honey.
2. Serve the oatmeal in small bowls with banana slices. Top with a dollop of yogurt, a sprinkle of pistachios and a little warm milk.

405 Cal, 7 g fat (saturated 1 g),
6 g fiber, 19 g protein, 67 g carbohydrate

mixed-grain oatmeal with berry compote

Serves 4   Preparation time: 10 minutes
Cooking time: 15 minutes (*pictured at left*)

3/4 cup rolled oats
3/4 cup rolled barley
1/4 cup roasted buckwheat
1/2 cup low fat milk, light soy milk
  or water
1/4 cup walnut pieces, chopped
2 tablespoons flaxseeds
2 tablespoons sunflower seeds
1 cup fresh or frozen mixed berries
low fat vanilla or soy yogurt, to serve

1. Place the oats, barley and buckwheat in a medium-sized saucepan with 3 cups water. Bring to a boil, then reduce the heat and simmer, stirring frequently, for 5 minutes or until creamy. Remove from heat and stir in the milk, walnuts, flaxseeds and sunflower seeds.
2. Place the berries in a small saucepan and gently heat until warmed and softened.
3. Spoon the oatmeal evenly into 4 bowls and served topped with a dollop of berry compote and a spoonful of yogurt.

363 Cal, 14 g fat (saturated 1 g),
5 g fiber, 10 g protein, 44 g carbohydrate

spiced fruit compote

Serves 4   Preparation time: 5 minutes
Cooking time: 15 minutes

⅔ cup dried apple rings, halved
⅓ cup dried apricots
⅓ cup pitted prunes
5 small (about 2½ oz) dried pears, halved
3 cardamom pods, flattened
2 whole cloves
1 cinnamon stick, broken
low fat natural yogurt, to serve

Place all ingredients (except yogurt) with 2 cups water in a medium-sized saucepan. Bring to the boil, then reduce heat, partially cover and simmer for 10–15 minutes, or until the fruit is soft. Serve warm or cold with yogurt. The compote will keep in an airtight container in the refrigerator for up to 1 week.

94 Cal, 0 g fat (saturated 0 g),
4 g fiber, 1 g protein, 21 g carbohydrate

stewed rhubarb and ginger

Serves 5   Preparation time: 10 minutes
Cooking time: 10 minutes

1 bunch rhubarb (1 lb untrimmed), ends trimmed,
   cut into ¾ in pieces
1¼ in piece fresh ginger, peeled and thinly sliced
2 tablespoons pure floral honey, pure maple syrup
   or rice syrup

Place all ingredients in a large heavy-based saucepan with 2 tablespoons water. Cover and bring to a simmer over medium–high heat. Cook, partially covered and stirring occasionally, for 6–7 minutes, or until rhubarb softens. Transfer to an airtight container to cool. It will store for 1 week if kept in the airtight container in the refrigerator. Remove ginger slices before serving.

52 Cal, 0 g fat (saturated 0 g),
2 g fiber, 1 g protein, 11 g carbohydrate

natural nutty muesli with stewed rhubarb and ginger

Makes about 10 cups (½ cup serve) Preparation time: 15 minutes

4 cups rolled oats

2 cups rye or barley flakes (or use
  extra oats)

½ cup pumpkin seeds

½ cup flaxseeds

⅔ cup sunflower seeds

⅔ cup slivered almonds

1¼ cups pecans, roughly chopped

1 cup dried apricots, chopped

¾ cup dried figs, chopped

low fat vanilla yogurt or light soy milk,
  to serve

Stewed Rhubarb and Ginger
  (see recipe page 78), or any fresh
  seasonal fruit, to serve

low fat milk or light soy milk, to serve

1. Place the rolled oats, rye flakes, pumpkin seeds, flaxseeds, sunflower seeds, almonds, pecans, apricots and figs in a large bowl. Toss well to combine.

2. Place ½ cup of this muesli in each of the 4 bowls, top with a dollop of yogurt or some milk and ¼ cup Stewed Rhubarb and Ginger. If you have added yogurt, add ¼ cup low fat milk or soy milk to moisten, and serve.

TIP

For a refreshing change, moisten the muesli at the end with a little sour cherry juice or pomegranate juice.

COOK'S TIP

To make toasted muesli, preheat the oven to 350°F. Combine the rolled oats, rye flakes, pumpkin seeds, flaxseeds and sunflower seeds. Divide among two large baking dishes. Bake, stirring frequently and turning the dishes around halfway through cooking, for 10–15 minutes, or until the oats are golden brown (take care they don't burn). Spread muesli onto a large plate or tray and set aside to cool. Now spread almonds and pecans over a baking tray and bake for 5–6 minutes, or until lightly toasted. Transfer to a large bowl and stir in remaining ingredients. The muesli will store for 1 month if kept in an airtight container.

298 Cal, 16 g fat (saturated 1 g),
5 g fiber, 8 g protein, 27 g carbohydrate

bircher muesli with mango and passionfruit

Serves 2 Preparation time: 5 minutes

Soaking time: overnight *(pictured at right)*

1 cup rolled oats
1 cup low fat milk or light soy milk
1 tablespoon pure floral honey, pure maple syrup or
   rice syrup
½ mango, flesh removed and cut into thin strips
2 passionfruit, pulp removed
4 strawberries, hulled, thinly sliced
low fat natural yogurt or soy yogurt,
   to serve, optional

1. The night before, place the oats and milk in a bowl, stir in the honey, cover and refrigerate overnight.
2. In the morning, divide the oat mixture between two serving bowls. Combine the mango, passionfruit and strawberries in a bowl, spoon over the oats, and serve.

COOK'S TIP
To make bircher muesli with apple, stir in 1 grated apple (with skin) once the muesli has soaked overnight.

387 Cal, 5 g fat (saturated 1 g),
7 g fiber, 18 g protein, 63 g carbohydrate

mixed-berry buttermilk pancakes

Serves 4 (makes 8) Preparation time: 10 minutes
Cooking time: 40 minutes *(pictured page 72)*

1½ cups stone-ground whole wheat
   self-rising flour
2 cups buttermilk
2 eggs
3 tablespoons pure floral honey or pure maple syrup
½ cup frozen blueberries
½ cup frozen raspberries
olive oil spray
low fat vanilla or soy yogurt, to serve, optional

1. Place the flour in a large bowl. In a separate bowl, whisk the buttermilk and eggs together. Add to the flour with 2 tablespoons of the honey, and whisk until combined. Stir in the frozen blueberries and raspberries.
2. Spray a large non-stick frying pan with oil and place over medium heat. Spoon ⅓ cup of the batter into the pan, spreading it out slightly, and cook for 2–3 minutes, or until golden underneath. Turn and cook for a further 2 minutes, or until the pancake has risen and is cooked through. Repeat to make 8 pancakes. Serve drizzled with honey.

433 Cal, 7 g fat (saturated 3 g),
9 g fiber, 18 g protein, 70 g carbohydrate

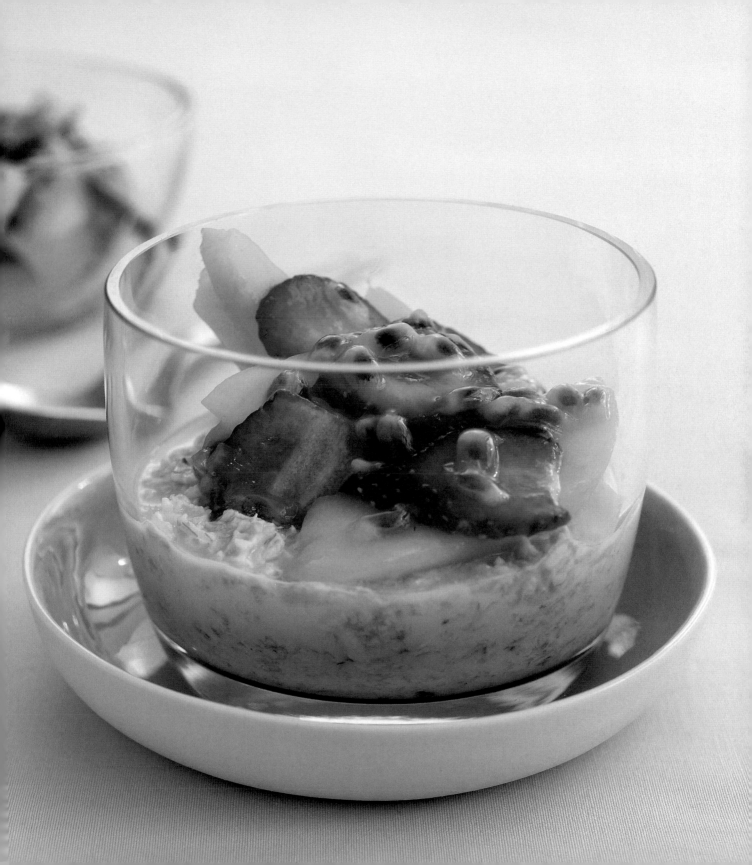

breakfast fried rice

Serves 4 Preparation time: 5 minutes   Cooking time: 10 minutes

1½ tablespoons olive oil

3 eggs, lightly beaten

3 scallions, trimmed, thinly sliced
   on the diagonal

3 ripe tomatoes, chopped

4½ cups cooked basmati rice

2–3 tablespoons reduced-sodium soy
   sauce

1. Heat 2 teaspoons of the oil and swirl around the wok to completely coat the sides. Add half of the egg mixture and swirl around to coat the inside of the wok. Cook for 2 minutes, or until set.

2. Carefully remove the cooked egg from the wok, and repeat with the remaining egg mixture. Roll up each omelet, cut into thin strips and set aside.

3. Heat the remaining oil in a wok over high heat. Add the scallion and tomato and cook for 1 minute. Add the rice and toss until heated through. Toss in soy sauce to taste, and serve immediately.

COOK'S TIP

If you don't have any leftover rice, cook 1⅓ cups of uncooked rice. To cool it quickly, spread the rice out over a large tray.

382 Cal, 11 g fat (saturated 2 g),
3 g fiber, 11 g protein, 56 g carbohydrate

corn and zucchini muffins

Serves 6   Preparation time: 15 minutes   Cooking time: 30 minutes   Cooling time: 15 minutes

2 cups stone-ground whole wheat
  self-rising flour
2 teaspoons baking powder
1½ cups fresh corn kernels (about 3
  small cobs)
2 (about 9 oz) zucchini, finely grated,
  moisture squeezed out
1 carrot (about 4½ oz), finely grated
⅓ cup finely grated parmesan
1½ cups buttermilk
2 tablespoons light olive oil
2 eggs

These muffins are best eaten on the day they are made.

1. Preheat oven to 350°F. Lightly grease a 6-cup large muffin pan.
2. Place the flour, baking powder, corn, zucchini, carrot and parmesan in a large bowl and mix well. In a separate bowl, whisk the buttermilk, oil and eggs together. Add to the dry ingredients and mix until just combined.
3. Spoon the mixture evenly among the muffin cups. Bake for 25–30 minutes, or until golden and a skewer inserted into the centers comes out clean. Set aside in the pan for 15 minutes before turning out. Serve warm or at room temperature.

402 Cal, 13 g fat (saturated 4 g), 9 g fiber, 16 g protein, 50 g carbohydrate

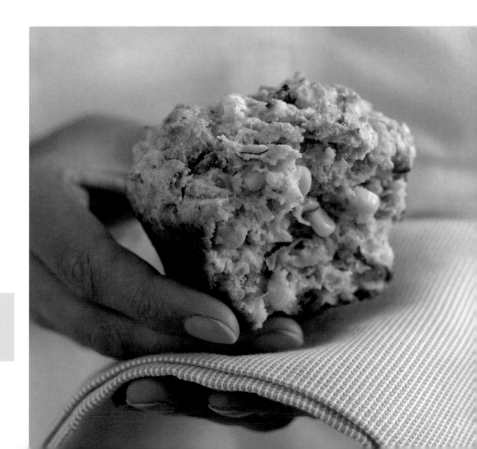

rice and cilantro fritters

Serves 4 (makes 16) Preparation time: 15 minutes Cooking time: 1 hour

1 cup medium-grain brown rice

½ red pepper, finely chopped

½ cup fresh corn kernels (about 1 small cob)

3 scallions, finely chopped

⅓ cup finely chopped fresh cilantro

2 tablespoons unbleached all-purpose flour

3 eggs, lightly whisked

salt and freshly ground black pepper

¼ cup olive oil

⅓ cup low fat natural yogurt, to serve

1 tablespoon sweet chili sauce, to serve

chopped cilantro, extra, to serve

1. Cook the rice in a medium-sized saucepan of boiling water, following package directions or until just tender. Drain well and set aside to cool.
2. Place the rice, pepper, corn, scallion and cilantro in a large bowl. Stir well to combine. Stir in the flour, add the eggs and mix until well combined. Season well, and stir. Use batter immediately.
3. Heat 1 tablespoon of oil in a large non-stick frying pan over medium heat. Add ¼ cup of the batter to the pan at a time, spreading it out slightly. Cook for 3–4 minutes each side, or until golden brown and set. Transfer to a plate lined with paper towels. Repeat with the remaining oil and batter to make 16 fritters, reheating the oil between each batch and stirring the batter to redistribute the egg.
4. Divide the fritters, in stacks, among 4 serving plates. Top each stack with 1 tablespoon of yogurt and 1 teaspoon of sweet chili sauce. Sprinkle with a little extra cilantro, and serve.

439 Cal, 20 g fat (saturated 4 g), 4 g fiber, 12 g protein, 51 g carbohydrate

grilled tomatoes and stuffed mushrooms

Serves 4   Preparation time: 15 minutes   Cooking time: 25 minutes

4 large vine-ripened tomatoes, halved
   horizontally
1½ tablespoons balsamic vinegar
1½ tablespoons extra-virgin olive oil
salt and freshly ground black pepper
1 clove garlic, crushed
8 large mushrooms, stems removed
7 oz low fat ricotta
2 tablespoons finely chopped fresh dill
2 tablespoons finely chopped parsley
1 teaspoon finely grated lemon rind
1 tablespoon fresh lemon juice
2¼ oz baby spinach or arugula leaves
4 thick slices grainy, low GI bread,
   toasted, to serve

1. Preheat the oven to 350°F. Line a baking tray with parchment paper.
2. Place the tomatoes, cut side up, on the tray, drizzle with 2 teaspoons each of the vinegar and oil and sprinkle with a little salt. Bake for 20 minutes, or until just tender.
3. Meanwhile, combine the remaining oil and the garlic. Brush the tops of the mushrooms with the garlic oil and place, stem side down, on a baking tray lined with baking paper. Bake for 20 minutes.
4. Place the ricotta in a bowl, and use a fork to break it up. Add the dill, parsley, lemon rind and lemon juice. Mix well, and season.
5. Turn the mushrooms over and fill with the ricotta mixture. Return to the oven for a further 5 minutes, or until filling is heated through.
6. Divide the spinach among 4 serving plates. Top with the mushrooms and tomatoes. Drizzle with a teaspoon of the remaining vinegar, and serve with toasted grainy bread.

255 Cal, 13 g fat (saturated 4 g),
5 g fiber, 12 g protein, 20 g carbohydrate

pancakes with tofu, basil and sun-dried tomato

Serves 4 (makes 8)   Preparation time: 15 minutes   Cooking time: 40 minutes

10½ oz silken tofu, drained

2 eggs

1 cup low fat soy milk

1 cup stone-ground whole wheat
  self-rising flour

½ cup buckwheat flour

1 tablespoon baking powder

½ cup sun-dried tomatoes, patted dry
  with paper towel, finely chopped

½ cup finely shredded basil

olive oil spray

2¼ oz baby arugula leaves

½ cup strips grilled pepper

1 tablespoon balsamic vinegar

1½ teaspoons flaxseed oil

salt and freshly ground black pepper

1. To make the pancakes, place the tofu in a bowl and use a fork to mash. Whisk in the eggs and soy milk. Sift in the whole wheat flour, buckwheat flour and baking powder, and mix until well combined. Stir in the sun-dried tomatoes and basil.

2. Spray a large non-stick frying pan with oil and place over medium heat. Drop ⅓ cup of the batter into the pan, spreading it out to about 6 in in diameter. Cook for 3 minutes, or until golden underneath. Turn and cook a further 2 minutes, or until the pancake has risen and is golden brown and cooked through. Repeat with the remaining batter to make 8 pancakes.

3. Place the arugula and grilled pepper in a bowl. Whisk the vinegar and flaxseed oil together, and season. Add to arugula mixture and toss to combine. Divide pancakes among serving plates, top with dressed arugula and pepper, and serve.

417 Cal, 12 g fat (saturated 2 g),
10 g fiber, 22 g protein, 51 g carbohydrate

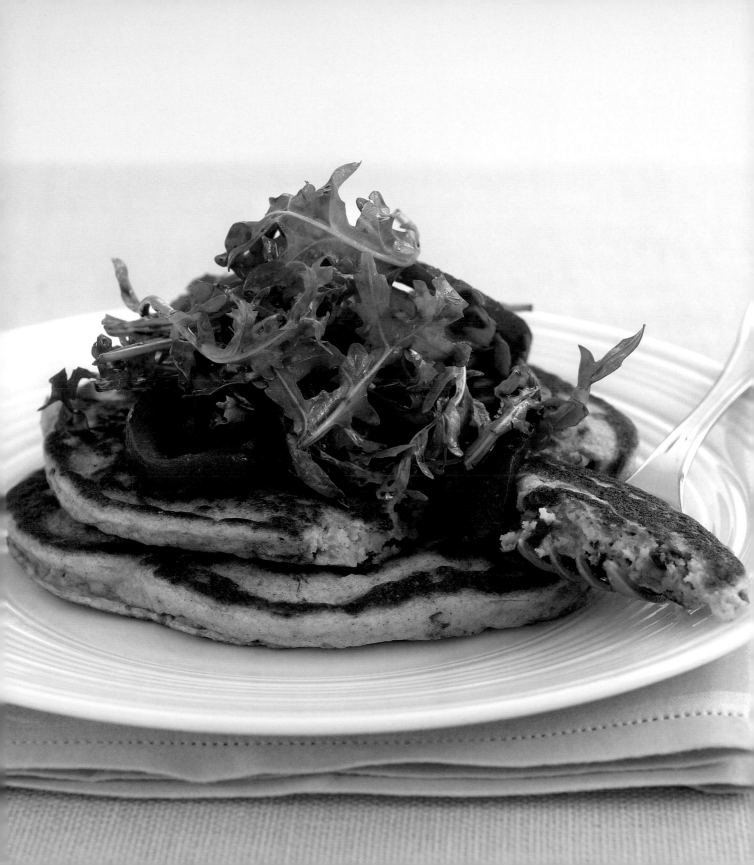

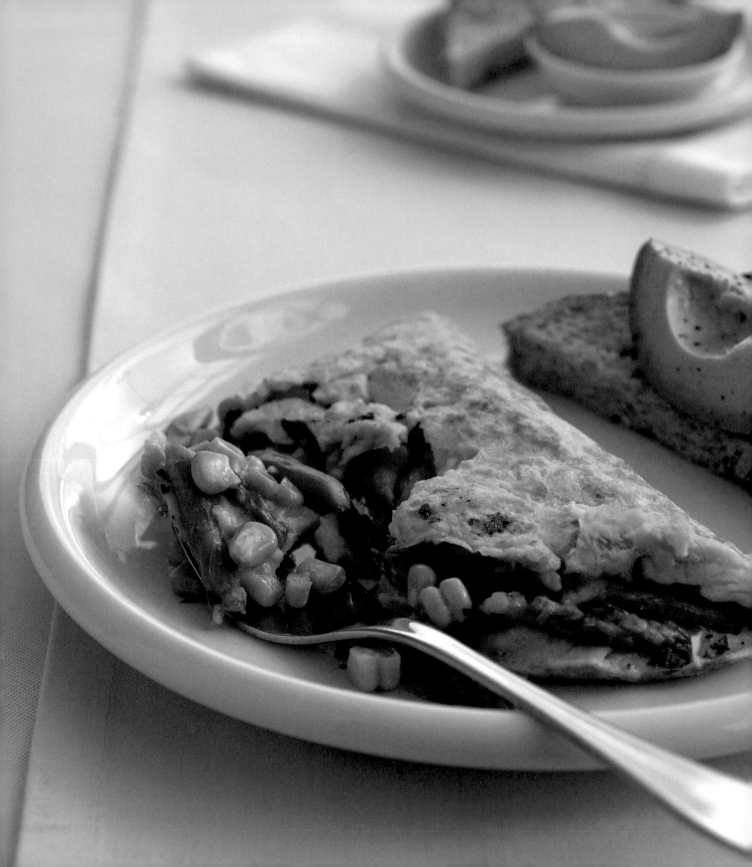

asparagus and corn omelet

Serves 2 Preparation time: 10 minutes   Cooking time: 10 minutes

1 tablespoon olive oil

1 bunch (5½ oz) asparagus, stalk ends
   trimmed, cut into ¾ in pieces

½ cup fresh corn kernels (about
   ½ large cob)

1 tablespoon finely chopped flat-leaf
   parsley

salt and freshly ground black pepper

4 eggs

2 tablespoons finely grated parmesan

2 slices grainy bread, toasted

¼ small avocado

1. Heat 2 teaspoons of the oil in a small, non-stick frying pan over medium–high heat. Add the asparagus and corn and cook for 2–3 minutes, or until vegetables are just tender. Remove to a bowl, stir in the parsley and season well.

2. Use a fork to whisk the eggs with 2 tablespoons of water. Heat 1 teaspoon of the remaining oil in the frying pan over medium heat. Pour in half of the egg mixture and cook for 3 minutes, or until almost set, using a fork to pull the cooked egg away from the edges and allow the uncooked egg to run to the edges.

3. Sprinkle half the asparagus and corn mixture, and half the parmesan, over half of the omelet and fold over to enclose. Lift out carefully and set aside.

4. Repeat with the remaining egg mixture and filling. Spread each toast with avocado and serve with the omelet.

TIP

If you have two small frying pans, you can cook both omelets at the same time.

COOK'S TIP

To make a pepper and mushroom omelet, replace the asparagus and corn with ½ small red pepper, finely chopped, and 3½ oz button mushrooms, thinly sliced. Increase cooking time for vegetables to 3–4 minutes. Replace parsley with chives, and continue from step 2.

446 Cal, 29 g fat (saturated 7 g),
4 g fiber, 22 g protein, 24 g carbohydrate

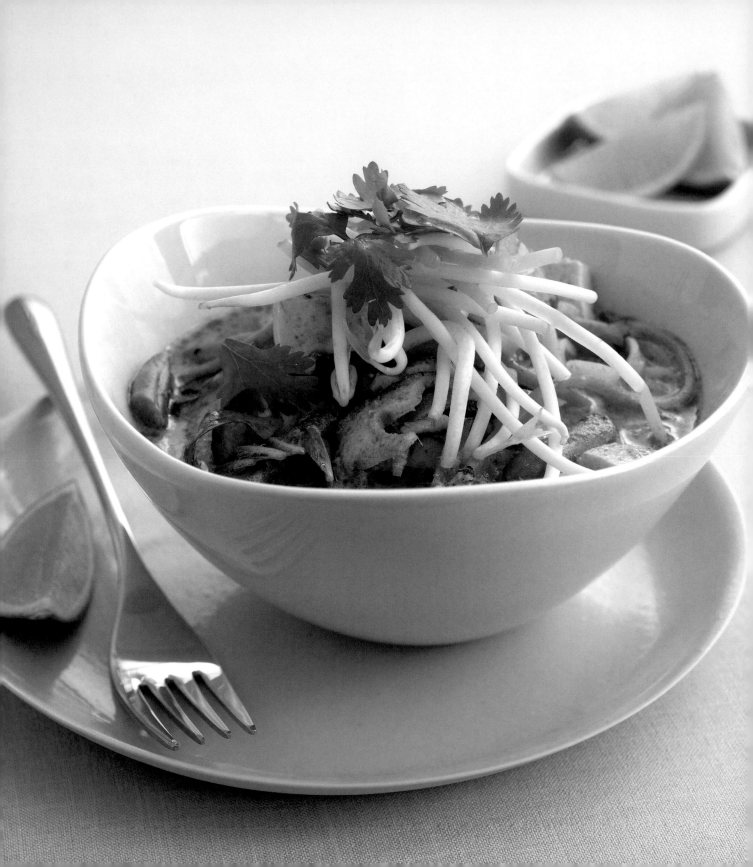

light meals, lunches and savory snacks

It is important to take a break and refuel properly at lunchtime.

A healthy, low GI lunch will help maintain energy and concentration

levels throughout the afternoon and reduce the temptation to snack on

something a little too indulgent later in the day. Lunch does not need to

be a big meal. In fact, if you find yourself feeling sleepy in the afternoon,

cut back on the carbs and boost the protein and vegetables at lunchtime.

vegetarian laksa

Serves 4   Preparation time: 15 minutes   Cooking time: 10 minutes (*pictured page 90*)

4½ oz dried rice-stick noodles

⅓ cup red curry paste

10½ oz firm tofu, patted dry with
  paper towel and cut into ½ inch
  cubes

2½ cups good-quality vegetable stock

9 fl oz can light coconut milk

1 large carrot, cut into short,
  thin sticks

3½ oz fresh shiitake mushrooms,
  thinly sliced

4½ oz green beans, diagonally sliced

3 baby bok choy, leaves separated,
  washed, shredded

1 tablespoon brown sugar

¾ cup bean sprouts

½ cup picked cilantro leaves

lime wedges, to serve

1. Cook the noodles in a large saucepan of boiling water for 2 minutes or until just tender. Drain well. Divide among 4 large serving bowls.

2. Heat a large wok over high heat. Add the curry paste and tofu and cook for 2 minutes. Add the stock and coconut milk and bring to a simmer. Add the carrot, mushrooms and beans and cook for 2 minutes. Add the bok choy and cook for a further 1 minute, or until just tender. Remove from the heat and stir in the sugar.

3. Divide the vegetables among the 4 serving bowls. Pour over the liquid evenly. Top with the bean sprouts and cilantro, and serve with the lime wedges.

397 Cal, 20 g fat (saturated 8 g),
8 g fiber, 17 g protein, 34 g carbohydrate

gazpacho with parmesan pumpernickel toasts

Serves 6   Preparation time: 20 minutes   Chilling time: 4 hours   Cooking time: 10 minutes

3 slices white sourdough, soaked in
½ cup water for 10 minutes, drained
and squeezed a little to remove
excess water
2 lb 4 oz very ripe vine-ripened
tomatoes, chopped
1 long green chile, deseeded
and chopped
2 Lebanese cucumbers, chopped
1 large red pepper, deseeded and
chopped
2 cloves garlic, peeled
1 cup picked basil leaves
1 cup picked flat-leaf parsley leaves
2 tablespoons extra-virgin olive oil
2 tablespoons balsamic vinegar
1 tablespoon caster sugar
salt and freshly ground black pepper
ice cubes, to serve
finely chopped cucumber and pepper,
extra, to serve

PARMESAN PUMPERNICKEL
TOASTS
4 slices pumpernickel bread
¼ cup finely grated parmesan

1. Place the sourdough, tomato, chile, cucumber, pepper, garlic, basil, parsley, oil, vinegar and sugar in a large food processor. Process until well combined. Add enough water (around 1½ cups) until you get the desired pouring consistency. Season well to taste. Transfer to a bowl or airtight container and refrigerate for 4 hours, or until well chilled.
2. Meanwhile, to make the Parmesan Pumpernickel Toasts, preheat oven to 350°F. Cut each slice of bread into 3 strips. Place on a baking tray lined with baking paper. Sprinkle parmesan evenly over bread. Bake for 8–10 minutes, or until parmesan is golden. Set aside to cool.
3. Serve the gazpacho, with a few ice cubes floating in it, with the Parmesan Pumpernickel Toasts, and bowls of chopped cucumber and pepper alongside.

227 Cal, 8 g fat (saturated 2 g),
7 g fiber, 7 g protein, 27 g carbohydrate

black bean soup

Serves 6 Preparation time: 30 minutes Cooking time: 1 hour

1 cup dried black beans,
  soaked overnight in cold water
1½ tablespoons olive oil
2 red onions, halved,
  thinly sliced
1 red pepper, chopped
1 green pepper, chopped
2 sticks celery, chopped
3 cloves garlic, crushed
2 dried bay leaves
2 teaspoons dried oregano
4 cups good-quality vegetable stock
2 tablespoons tomato paste
¾ cup fresh corn kernels
  (about 1 large cob)
salt and freshly ground black pepper

1. Rinse soaked black beans under cold water, drain, and set aside.
2. Heat the oil in a large heavy-based saucepan over medium heat. Add the onion and cook for 6–7 minutes, or until soft. Add the peppers, celery and garlic and cook for a further 4 minutes. Stir in the black beans, bay leaves, oregano, stock and tomato paste with 2 cups water, and bring to a simmer. Simmer, partially covered, for 30 minutes, then stir in the corn and cook for a further 15 minutes, or until beans are tender.
3. Remove bay leaves from soup, season to taste, and serve.

624 Cal, 23 g fat (saturated 6 g),
10 g fiber, 24 g protein, 76 g carbohydrate

bean and corn burritos

Serves 4   Preparation time: 20 minutes   Cooking time: 25 minutes

1 tablespoon olive oil
1 red onion, halved,
  thinly sliced
¾ cup fresh corn kernels (about 1
  large cob)
1 red pepper, thinly sliced
1 green pepper, thinly sliced
2 teaspoons ground cilantro
2 teaspoons mild paprika
1 teaspoon ground cumin
½ teaspoon chili powder
1 – 14 oz can Italian chopped
  tomatoes
1¼ cups cooked red kidney beans
2 tablespoons tomato paste
½ cup good-quality vegetable stock
¼ cup finely chopped cilantro
10 corn tortillas
1 ripe avocado
1 tablespoon fresh lemon juice
salt and freshly ground black pepper
low fat natural yogurt, to serve

1. Heat the oil in a large non-stick frying pan over medium heat. Add the onion, corn and peppers and cook for 5 minutes, or until vegetables soften. Add the ground cilantro, paprika, cumin and chili powder. Cook, stirring, for 1 minute.
2. Add the tomatoes, kidney beans, tomato paste and stock to the pan. Stir well. Bring to a simmer. Simmer, uncovered, for 10 minutes. Remove from heat and stir in the cilantro.
3. Meanwhile, preheat oven to 350°F. Wrap the tortillas in foil and warm in the oven for 5 minutes.
4. Mash the flesh of the avocado with the lemon juice, and season. Serve tortillas topped with the bean mixture, avocado and yogurt.

451 Cal, 21 g fat (saturated 4 g),
12 g fiber, 16 g protein, 44 g carbohydrate

spicy moroccan chickpea and lentil soup

Serves 6 Preparation time: 20 minutes   Cooking time: 50 minutes

1 tablespoon olive oil
1 large onion, finely chopped
3 cloves garlic, crushed
1 in piece fresh ginger, finely grated
3 teaspoons ground cilantro
2 teaspoons ground cumin
½ teaspoon chili powder
½ teaspoon saffron threads soaked
  in 2 tablespoons boiling water
14 oz can Italian chopped tomatoes
4 cups good-quality vegetable stock
1 cup red lentils, rinsed well
2⅔ cups cooked chickpeas, drained
⅓ cup chopped cilantro
⅓ cup chopped flat-leaf parsley,
  plus extra, to serve
salt and freshly ground black pepper
low fat natural yogurt, to serve

1. Heat the oil in a large, heavy-based saucepan over medium heat. Add the onion and cook, stirring occasionally, for 6–7 minutes, or until soft. Add the garlic, ginger, cilantro, cumin and chili powder, and cook, stirring, for 1 minute.
2. Add the saffron with its soaking liquid, tomatoes, stock, lentils and 4 cups water to the pan. Cover and bring to a simmer. Simmer, uncovered, for 30 minutes. Add chickpeas and cook for a further 10 minutes.
3. Remove the pan from the heat and stir in the cilantro and parsley. Season to taste, top with a dollop of yogurt, and sprinkle with extra chopped parsley.

TIP
You can replace the chickpeas with soy beans or any kind of white bean, if you prefer.

292 Cal, 7 g fat (saturated 1 g),
2 g fiber, 19 g protein, 33 g carbohydrate

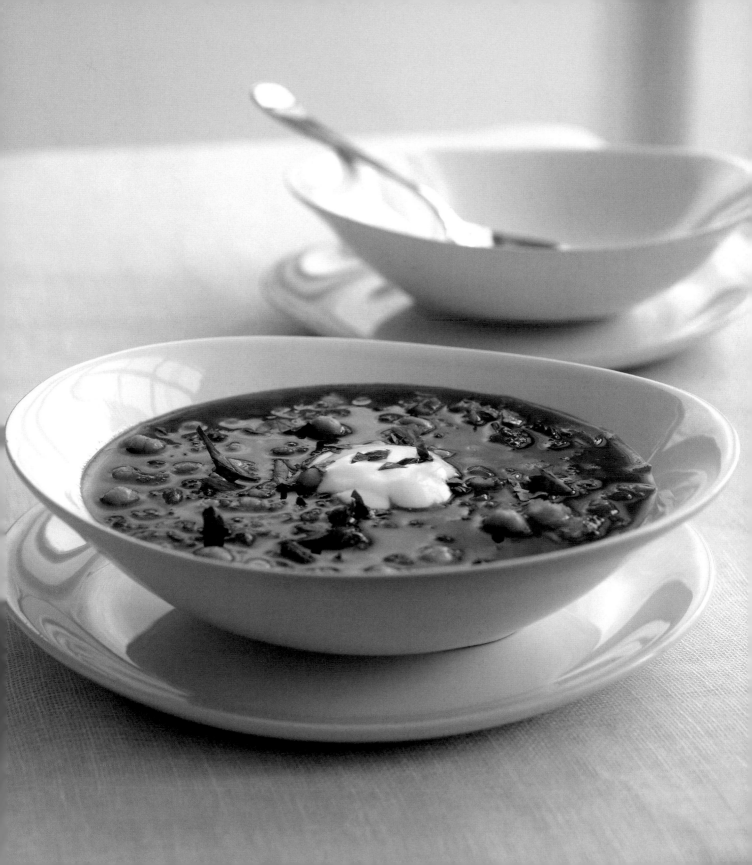

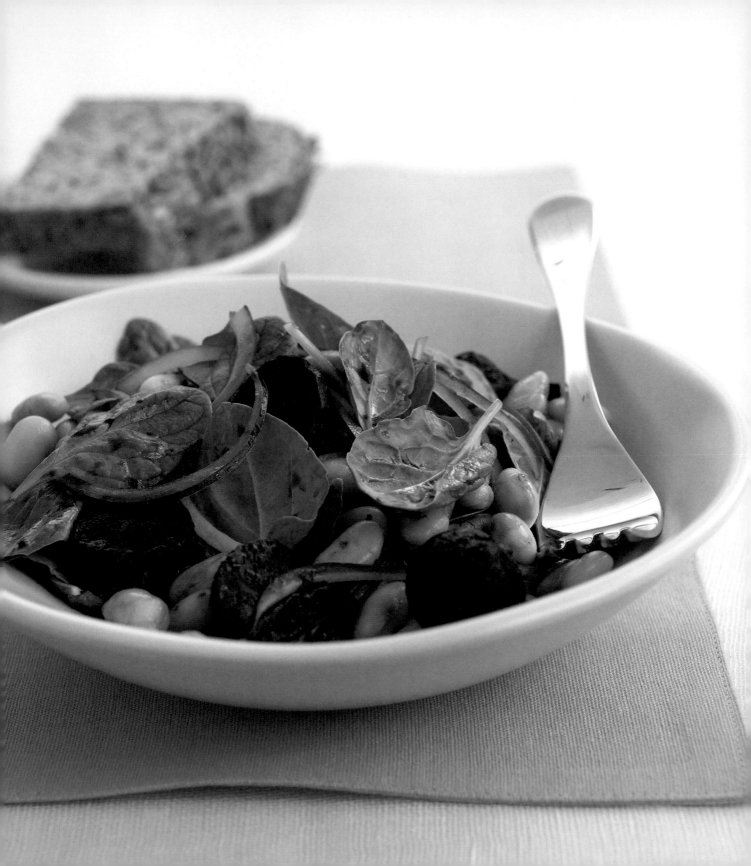

roasted beet and white-bean salad with balsamic dressing

Serves 4   Preparation time: 10 minutes   Cooking time: 1½–2 hours

1 bunch (1 lb 5 oz) beets
4½ oz baby spinach leaves
3 cups cooked white beans
1 red onion, halved, thinly sliced
4 thick slices wholegrain or rye bread,
  to serve

BALSAMIC DRESSING
1½ tablespoons balsamic vinegar
2 teaspoons flaxseed oil
1 clove garlic, crushed
salt and freshly ground black pepper

1. Preheat oven to 350°F.
2. Trim off the beet leaves, leaving about 1¼ in of the tops intact. (Do not trim bases, as this will cause the beets to bleed and lose its color.) Wrap beets in a large piece of foil and place on a baking tray. Roast for 1½–2 hours, or until tender. Set aside to cool. Once cool, put on rubber gloves and peel the beet. Cut into thin wedges.
3. Place the spinach leaves, beans and onion in a bowl. Toss to combine. Add the beet and toss gently to combine.
4. To make the Balsamic Dressing, place the vinegar, oil and garlic in a small small pitcher. Whisk well to combine, and season to taste.
5. Pour the dressing over the salad and toss to combine. Serve immediately with the bread.

TIP
You can replace the white beans with chickpeas or soy beans, if desired.

341 Cal, 4 g fat (saturated 1 g),
17 g fiber, 18 g protein, 51 g carbohydrate

individual frittatas with pepper, sweet potato, baby peas and feta

Serves 6   Preparation time: 15 minutes   Cooking time: 30–35 minutes   Cooling time: 10 minutes

1 tablespoon extra-virgin olive oil

1 red onion, halved, thinly sliced

1 red pepper, cut into short, thin strips

10½ oz orange sweet potato, cut into
  ½ in pieces

1 clove garlic, crushed

1 cup frozen baby green peas

⅓ cup semi-dried tomatoes, finely
  chopped

3½ oz low fat feta, crumbled

olive oil spray

7 eggs

½ cup low fat milk or soy milk

salt and freshly ground black pepper

dressed salad leaves, to serve

1. Heat the oil in a large, non-stick frying pan over medium–high heat. Add the onion, pepper, sweet potato and garlic. Cook, stirring often, for 5 minutes. Add the peas and cook for 3 minutes. Remove from the heat and set aside to cool a little. Stir in the semi-dried tomatoes and feta.

2. Preheat oven to 375°F. Spray a large 6-cup muffin pan with oil. Whisk together the eggs and milk, and season. Divide the vegetables among the muffin pan cups. Pour the egg mixture evenly over the vegetables.

3. Bake for 20–25 minutes, or until frittatas are set and lightly golden. Set aside in the pan for 10 minutes before turning out. Serve warm with dressed salad leaves.

251 Cal, 12 g fat (saturated 4 g),
5 g fiber, 17 g protein, 16 g carbohydrate

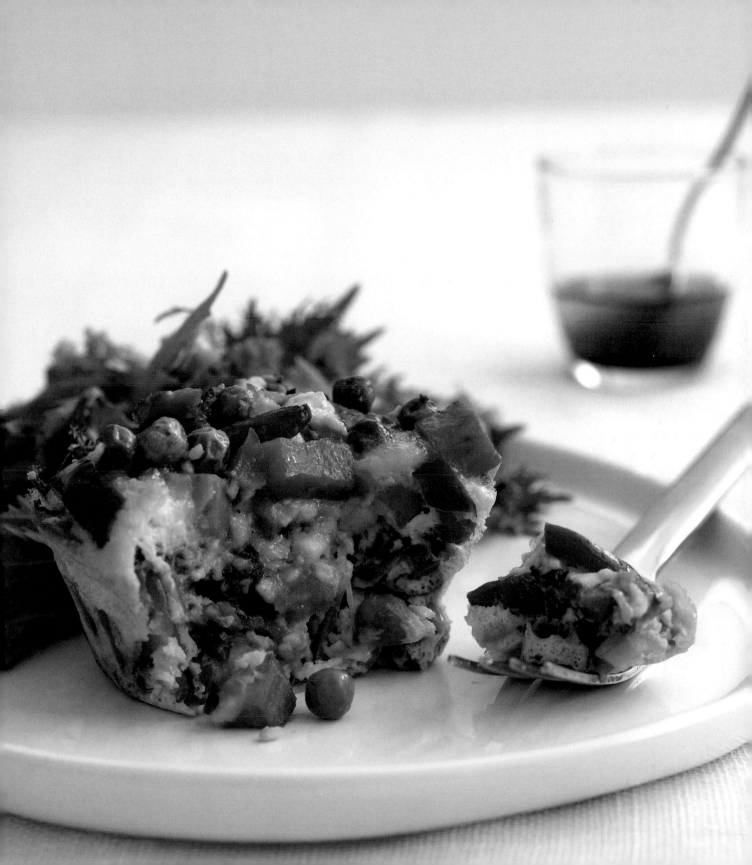

herb and garlic baked ricotta

Serves 8   Preparation time: 5 minutes   Standing time: overnight   Cooking time: 1 hour 20 minutes

2 lb 4 oz whole round of
 low fat ricotta
2 tablespoons extra-virgin olive oil
salt and freshly ground black pepper
1½ tablespoons finely chopped
 flat-leaf parsley
1½ tablespoons finely chopped basil
1 clove garlic, crushed

This ricotta is wonderful served as part of an antipasto platter, on sliced rye bread topped with sliced vine-ripened tomatoes, or simply on its own.

1. Place the ricotta in a large sieve over a bowl. Cover with plastic wrap and refrigerate overnight to allow any excess liquid to drain out.
2. Preheat oven to 400°F. Line a baking tray with baking paper.
3. Place the ricotta on the tray. Brush one tablespoon of the oil over the ricotta and season well. Bake for 40 minutes, brushing occasionally with the oil, until the edges and top start to change color. Reduce oven temperature to 315°F.
4. Meanwhile, combine the parsley, basil, garlic and remaining oil in a bowl, and brush over the ricotta. Bake, brushing twice with the oil, for a further 30–40 minutes, or until lightly golden all over. Set aside to cool completely.
5. Serve at room temperature. The ricotta can be kept in an airtight container in the refrigerator for up to 1 week.

199 Cal, 15 g fat (saturated 8 g),
0 g fiber, 13 g protein, 3 g carbohydrate

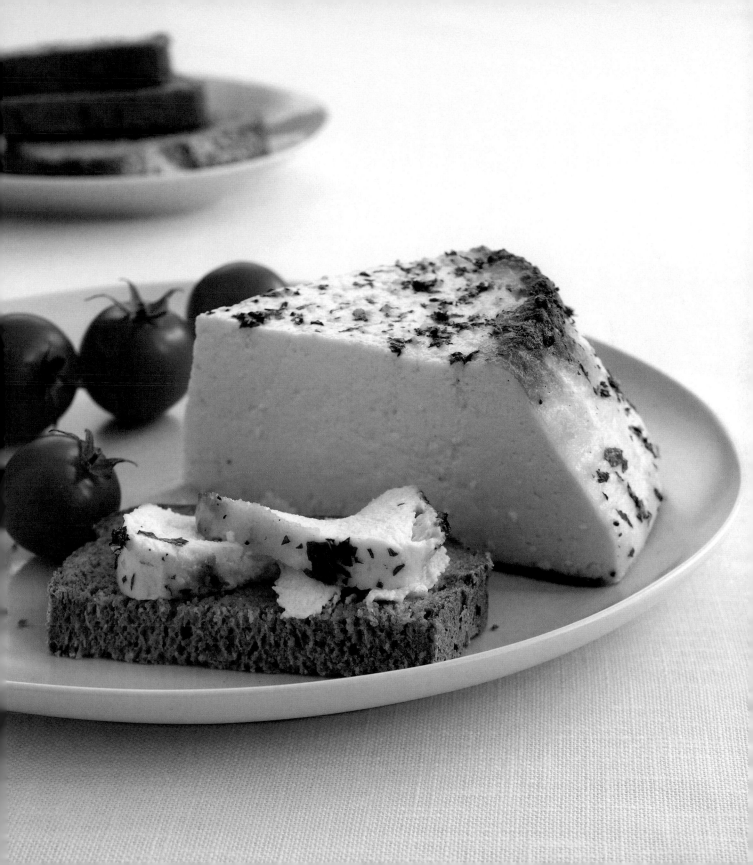

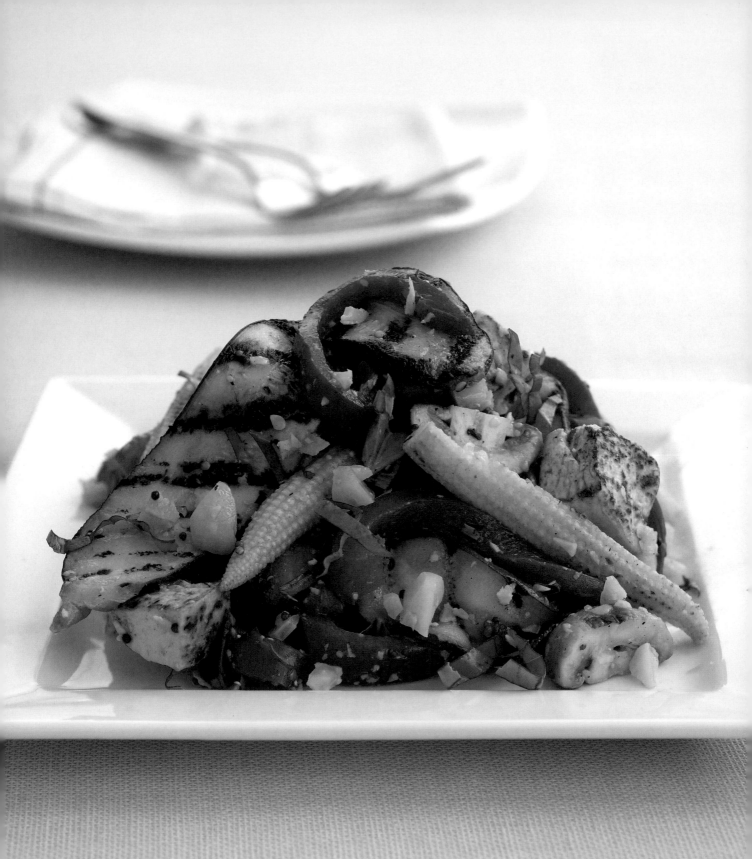

grilled vegetable and tofu salad

Serves 4 Preparation time: 20 minutes Cooking time: 20 minutes

2 red peppers, quartered, deseeded

2 zucchini, thinly sliced lengthways

3 baby (finger) eggplants, thinly sliced
  lengthways

7 oz whole button mushrooms, stems
  trimmed, halved

4½ oz baby corn, halved lengthways

2½ tablespoons olive oil

13 oz firm tofu, patted dry with paper
  towel, cut into ½ in thick slices

3½ oz unsalted macadamias,
  chopped

1 cup finely shredded basil

2 tablespoons white-wine or red-wine
  vinegar

1 tablespoon wholegrain mustard

salt and freshly ground black pepper

1. Preheat a barbecue grill and flat plate on medium–high. Place the pepper, zucchini, eggplant, mushrooms and corn in a large bowl. Add 2 teaspoons of the oil and toss to coat.

2. Place the pepper, skin side down, on the grill and cook for 3–4 minutes each side, or until the skin starts to blacken. Transfer to a bowl, cover with a tea towel and set aside to cool. Place the zucchini and eggplant on the grill and cook for 2–3 minutes each side, or until just tender. Transfer to a separate bowl. Place the mushrooms and corn on the flat plate. Cook, turning occasionally, for 3–4 minutes, or until cooked. Transfer to the bowl of vegetables. Brush tofu with 1 tablespoon of the remaining oil. Place on the grill and cook for 3–4 minutes each side, or until light golden. Cut into strips and add to vegetables.

3. Once the pepper is cool, peel away the skin and cut the flesh into thin strips. Add to the other cooked vegetables, along with the macadamias and basil. Toss to combine. In a separate bowl, whisk together the remaining oil, vinegar and mustard, and season well. Add to the vegetables and toss to combine. Serve.

374 Cal, 27 g fat (saturated 4 g),
8 g fiber, 18 protein, 12 g carbohydrate

balsamic barley salad with pepper, corn, zucchini and mushrooms

Serves 6   Preparation time: 20 minutes   Cooking time: 35 minutes

¾ cup pearl barley
1 corn cob, lightly steamed,
  kernels removed
1 zucchini, steamed until al dente,
  chopped
1 yellow pepper, deseeded, chopped
1 red pepper, deseeded, chopped
1 Lebanese cucumber, quartered
  lengthwise, deseeded, chopped
½ cup semi-dried tomatoes,
  roughly chopped
8 button mushrooms, stems removed,
  roughly chopped
3 spring onions, chopped
¼ cup finely chopped fresh dill

BALSAMIC DRESSING
2 tablespoons red-wine vinegar
2 tablespoons balsamic vinegar
3 tablespoons olive oil
freshly ground black pepper

1. Cook barley in a large saucepan of salted boiling water for 35 minutes, or until al dente. Drain in a colander, rinse and set aside to cool.
2. To make the Balsamic Dressing, whisk together all the dressing ingredients.
3. In a salad bowl, combine the barley with the remaining ingredients, toss with the dressing, and serve.

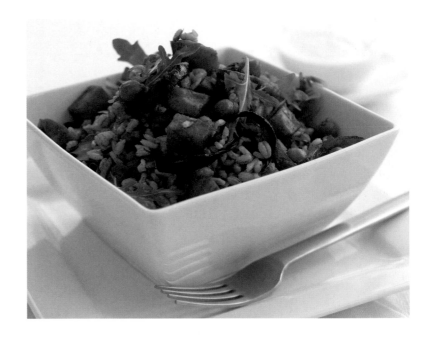

256 Cal, 11 g fat (saturated 2 g),
8 g fiber, 6 g protein, 28 g carbohydrate

roasted vegetable couscous

Serves 4 Preparation time: 20 minutes Cooking time: 45 minutes

2 zucchini, cut into about 1¼ in pieces

1 eggplant, cut into 1¼ in pieces

1 large red pepper, cut into 1¼ in pieces

9 oz orange sweet potato, peeled and cut into 1¼ in pieces

2 red onions, cut into thin wedges

1 leek, cut into 1¼ in lengths

1½ tablespoons picked fresh rosemary leaves

3 tablespoons olive oil

2⅔ cups cooked chickpeas or butter beans

1 – 9 oz punnet cherry tomatoes

3 cloves garlic, crushed

2 tablespoons pure floral honey or pure maple syrup

1 cup couscous

1 cup good-quality vegetable stock

½ cup finely chopped flat-leaf parsley

juice and finely grated rind of 1 lemon

salt and freshly ground black pepper

1. Preheat oven to 425°F. Line two roasting pans with baking paper.

2. Place the zucchini, eggplant, pepper, sweet potato, onion, leek and rosemary in a large bowl. Add 2 tablespoons of the oil. Toss well to combine. Divide vegetables among the roasting pans and roast, turning pans around halfway through cooking, for 30 minutes, or until vegetables are almost tender.

3. Add the chickpeas, tomatoes and garlic to the vegetables, and toss to combine. Drizzle 1 tablespoon of honey over each tray. Roast for a further 15 minutes, or until vegetables are golden and tender.

4. Meanwhile, place the couscous in a heatproof bowl. Place the stock in a small saucepan and bring to the boil. Pour over the couscous. Set aside for 3–4 minutes, or until liquid is absorbed. Use a fork to separate the grains. Stir in the parsley, lemon juice and lemon rind.

5. Transfer the roasted vegetables to a large serving bowl. Add the couscous mixture, toss well to combine, season well and serve.

613 Cal, 18 g fat (saturated 3 g),
14 g fiber, 20 g protein, 84 g carbohydrate

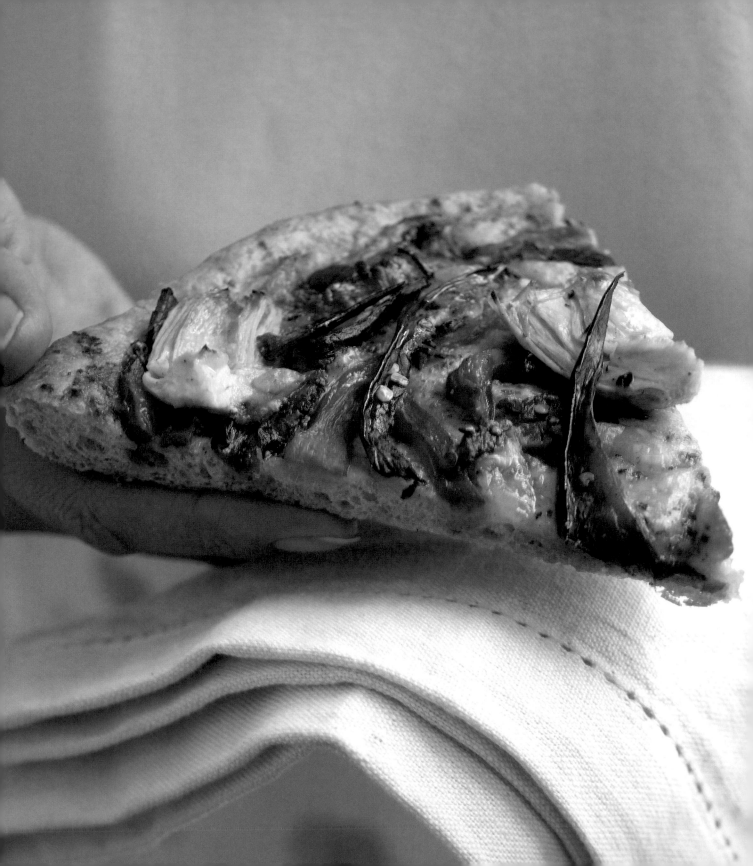

caramelized onion and goat cheese pizza, and grilled vegetable pizza

Serves 4 Preparation time: 20 minutes Standing time: 1 hour Cooking time: 40–50 minutes

1½ cups stone-ground whole wheat all-purpose flour

¼ oz sachet dried yeast

1 teaspoon salt

CARAMELIZED ONION AND GOAT CHEESE TOPPING

2 tablespoons olive oil

1 lb 10 oz red onions, halved, thinly sliced

2 tablespoons picked thyme leaves

2 cloves garlic, crushed

1 tablespoon brown sugar

1 tablespoon balsamic vinegar

2¼ oz goat cheese, crumbled

GRILLED VEGETABLE TOPPING

2 tablespoons basil pesto

3½ oz grilled pepper, patted dry with paper towel, cut into thin strips

2½ oz drained marinated artichoke hearts, cut into thin wedges

2½ oz grilled eggplant, patted dry with paper towel, cut into thin strips

2¼ oz bocconcini, thinly sliced

¼ cup picked basil leaves, to serve

1. To make the pizza dough, place the flour, yeast and salt in a bowl. Add ¾ cup lukewarm water and use a flat-bladed knife to mix until just combined. Turn out onto a lightly floured surface and knead until smooth. Place in a lightly oiled bowl, cover with plastic wrap and set aside in a warm place for 1 hour.

2. Meanwhile, to make the caramelized onions, heat the oil in a large, non-stick frying pan over medium heat. Add the onion, thyme and garlic, and stir to coat. Reduce heat to medium–low and cook, stirring occasionally, for 25–30 minutes, or until the onions are very soft. Add the sugar and vinegar, and increase the heat to high. Cook for a further 5 minutes, or until the onions start to caramelize. Set aside to cool completely.

3. Preheat oven to 450°F. Lightly grease two 11-inch round pizza trays.

4. Use your fist to pound the dough. Divide into two. Roll one portion out and use it to line one tray. Repeat with the remaining dough. Spread the caramelized onions over one of the bases, and sprinkle over the goat cheese. Spread the second base with the pesto. Top with the pepper, artichoke, eggplant and bocconcini.

5. Bake the pizzas, turning the trays halfway through cooking, for 15–20 minutes, or until the tops are golden and the bases are crisp. Sprinkle the grilled vegetable pizza with basil leaves, before serving.

Caramelized onion and goat cheese:
293 Cal, 12 g fat (saturated 3 g),
7 g fiber, 9 g protein, 34 g carbohydrate

Grilled vegetable:
375 Cal, 14 g fat (saturated 5 g),
10 g fiber, 17 g protein, 40 g carbohydrate

red lentil dahl with spiced basmati rice

Serves 4   Preparation time: 15 minutes   Standing time: 20 minutes   Cooking time: 30 minutes

1 cup red lentils
1 tablespoon olive oil
1 onion, finely chopped
1 clove garlic, crushed
1 – 1¼ in piece fresh ginger, peeled
   and finely grated
2 teaspoons ground cilantro
1 teaspoon ground cumin
1 teaspoon ground turmeric
½ teaspoon chili powder
3½ cups good-quality vegetable stock
salt and freshly ground black pepper
1 tablespoon fresh lemon juice
1 cup cilantro, roughly chopped
lime wedges, to serve

SPICED BASMATI RICE
1¼ cups basmati rice
1 tablespoon olive oil
1 tablespoon sesame seeds
2 teaspoons brown mustard seeds
2 teaspoons cumin seeds
1 cinnamon stick, broken
1 dried red chile
1¾ cups good-quality vegetable stock
⅓ cup roasted unsalted peanuts, finely
   chopped

1. To make the dahl, place the lentils in a sieve and rinse under cold running water until the water runs clear. Heat the oil in a large heavy-based saucepan over medium heat. Add the onion and garlic and cook for 6–7 minutes, or until the onion softens. Add the ginger, ground cilantro, cumin, turmeric and chili powder. Cook, stirring, for 1 minute. Stir in the lentils and stock. Cover and bring to a simmer. Simmer, uncovered, for 20–25 minutes, or until the lentils are soft and the mixture thickens. Season to taste. Stir in the lemon juice and cilantro leaves.

2. Meanwhile, to make the Spiced Basmati Rice, place rice in a bowl and cover with plenty of cold water. Set aside for 20 minutes, then rinse and drain well. Heat the oil in a medium-sized saucepan over medium heat. Add all the seeds, the cinnamon and the chile. Cook, stirring, for 1 minute. Remove cinnamon stick. Stir in the rice and stock. Cover and bring to a simmer. Reduce heat to low and cook, covered, without stirring, for 12 minutes. Remove pan from heat and set aside, covered, for 5 minutes. Add the peanuts and use a fork to separate the rice grains.

3. Serve the dahl with the Spiced Basmati Rice, and accompanied by lime wedges.

622 Cal, 20 g fat (saturated 3 g),
11 g fiber, 27 g protein, 78 g carbohydrate

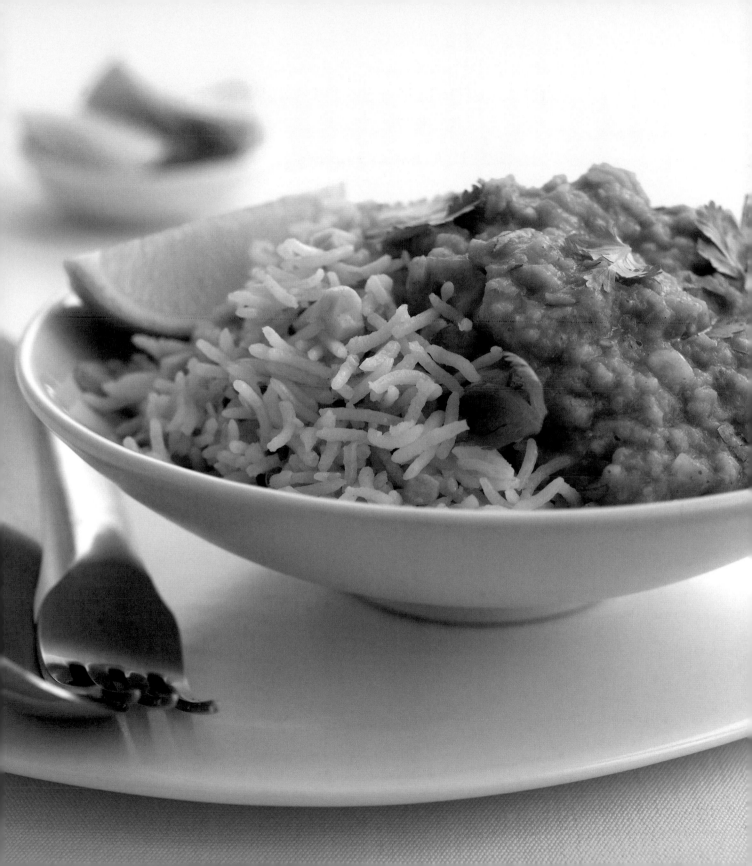

tofu, avocado and cucumber sushi

Serves 4   Preparation time: 20 minutes   Marinating time: 4 hours   Cooking time: 15 minutes (plus cooling time)

3½ oz firm tofu, cut into 2 slices, then
  cut again in half lengthways
2 tablespoons reduced-sodium soy
  sauce
2 tablespoons mirin
1 clove garlic, crushed
1 cup sushi (koshihikari) rice
⅓ cup sushi seasoning
4 sheets toasted nori
½ avocado, thinly sliced
1 Lebanese cucumber, seeds removed,
  cut into short strips
pickled ginger (optional)
soy sauce, extra, to serve
wasabi, to serve

1. Place the tofu in a small dish. Combine the soy sauce, mirin and garlic in a separate small dish. Pour sauce over the tofu, cover and place in the refrigerator to marinate for at least 4 hours.
2. Place the rice in a sieve and rinse under cold running water until the water runs clear. Place the rice in a medium-sized saucepan with 2 cups water. Bring to a simmer over medium heat. Cover, reduce heat to low, and cook for 12 minutes. Remove from heat and set aside, covered, for 5 minutes. Add the sushi seasoning and stir gently to combine. Spread over a tray and set aside to cool.
3. Place one sheet of nori, rough side up and with one of the long ends closest to you, on a clean surface. Using wet hands, place a quarter of the rice on the nori sheet, and pat down to cover the sheet, leaving 1½ in at the top of the sheet. Press the rice firmly down on the sheet.
4. Drain tofu from marinade. Place a piece of the tofu and a few slices of the avocado and cucumber on the sheet, about 1¼ in from the bottom, closest to you. Top with a little pickled ginger, if using. Starting from the end closest to you, roll up firmly. Repeat with remaining nori, rice and fillings. Using a wet knife, cut the rolls into thick slices.
5. Mix a little soy sauce and wasabi together, to taste. Serve sushi with soy and wasabi mixture.

303 Cal, 9 g fat (saturated 2 g),
2 g fiber, 9 g protein, 45 g carbohydrate

fennel, leek and bean barley pilaf

Serves 4   Preparation time: 15 minutes   Cooking time: 50 minutes

1 tablespoon olive oil

1 leek, trimmed and finely chopped

1 small bulb fennel, trimmed, finely
   chopped

1 clove garlic, crushed

½ teaspoon fennel seeds, lightly
   roasted, crushed

4 oz button mushrooms, sliced

1 corn cob, kernels removed

1 cup pearl barley

2 cups hot vegetable stock

5½ oz green beans, trimmed, sliced

salt and freshly ground
   black pepper

2 tablespoons chopped parsley

¼ cup slivered almonds,
   lightly toasted, to serve

Both fennel and fennel seeds have been added to this dish for extra flavor. Any variety of vegetables can be used.

1. Heat the oil in a large heavy-based saucepan, add the leek and fennel and cook over medium–low heat, stirring occasionally, for 6–7 minutes, or until leek is soft. Add the garlic and fennel seeds and cook, stirring, for 1 minute more.

2. Increase the heat to medium–high. Add the mushrooms and corn and cook, stirring, for 2 minutes. Add the barley and stock, stir to combine and bring to the boil. Reduce the heat to low, cover and simmer, stirring occasionally, for 35–40 minutes, or until the barley is almost tender and all the stock absorbed.

3. Add the green beans, and season. Cook for 3 minutes more, then mix in the parsley. Serve sprinkled with the almonds.

319 Cal, 11 g fat (saturated 1 g),
11 g fiber, 11 g protein, 39 g carbohydrate

vietnamese rice-paper rolls

Makes 12 Preparation time: 20 minutes

12 – 8½ in round rice papers
1 Lebanese cucumber, cut into short,
   thin sticks
1 small red pepper, cut into short,
   thin sticks
1 large carrot, cut into short,
   thin sticks
1 small avocado, cut into short,
   thin slices
1¾ oz snow pea sprouts, ends
   trimmed
¾ cup picked cilantro leaves
¾ cup picked mint leaves
⅓ cup unsalted roasted peanuts, finely
   chopped

DIPPING SAUCE
3 tablespoons sweet chili sauce
1½ tablespoons soy sauce
3 tablespoons fresh lime juice

These rice-paper rolls can be made a few hours in advance. Simply cover with damp paper towels, then plastic wrap, and refrigerate.

1. To make the Dipping Sauce, combine all sauce ingredients in a bowl. Set aside.
2. Place all the ingredients for the rice-paper rolls on a bench. Half-fill a large bowl with warm water. Dip one wrapper in the water for 20 seconds, or until it is just soft. Drain off excess water and place on a clean surface. Place a few pieces of each of the remaining ingredients on the wrapper, about 1¼ in in from the base. Fold up the bottom of the wrapper. Fold in the sides and roll up to enclose the filling. Place on a tray and cover with damp paper towels. Repeat with the remaining wrappers and filling ingredients.
3. Serve rice-paper rolls with the Dipping Sauce.

92 Cal, 6 g fat (saturated 1 g),
2 g fiber, 3 g protein, 5 g carbohydrate

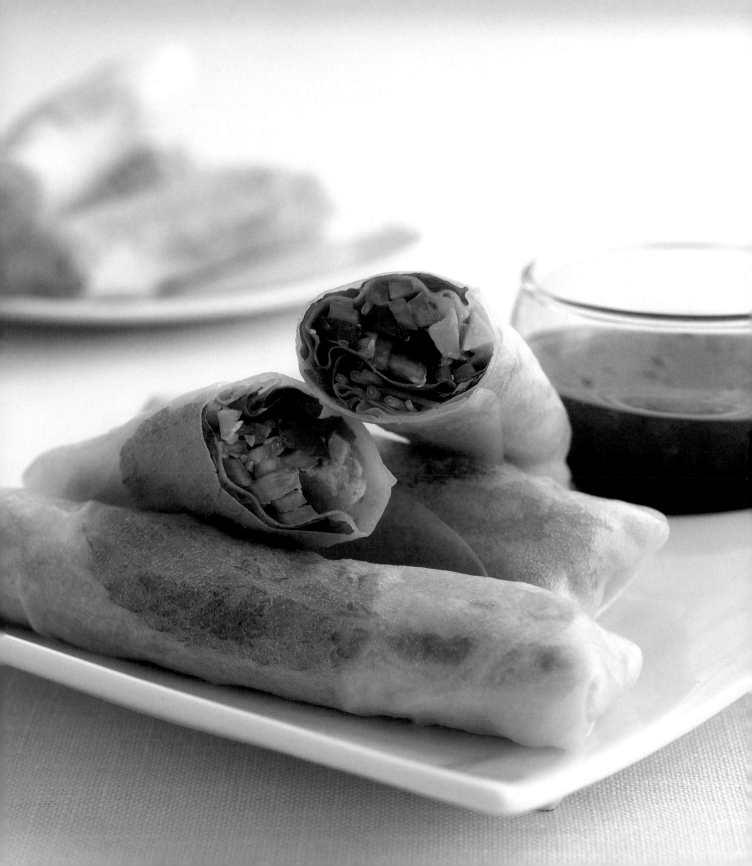

avocado, pickled ginger and tofu soba-noodle salad

Serves 4   Preparation: 15 minutes   Cooking time: 5 minutes

7 oz dried soba noodles

1 teaspoon sesame oil

5½ oz snow peas, trimmed, halved
   diagonally

7 oz marinated tofu (such as teriyaki),
   thinly sliced

1 Lebanese cucumber, halved, thinly
   sliced diagonally

2 tablespoons pickled ginger,
   thinly sliced

2½ oz baby spinach leaves

½ cup picked cilantro leaves

1 avocado, chopped, lemon juice
   squeezed over (to prevent
   discoloring)

3 spring onions, trimmed, sliced
   diagonally

¼ cup) lightly toasted cashews,
   roughly chopped

DRESSING

2 tablespoons mirin

3 tablespoons light soy sauce

1 teaspoon sesame oil

pinch Superfine sugar

This soba-noodle salad is light and refreshing, with clean Japanese flavors. It takes just minutes to prepare, using pre-marinated tofu available from supermarkets. Mirin is sweet Japanese cooking wine and is available from the Asian section of supermarkets.

1. To make the dressing, place all dressing ingredients in a small bowl, and stir to dissolve the sugar. Set aside.
2. Cook the soba noodles in a large saucepan of lightly salted boiling water according to package instructions, or until al dente. Rinse under cold running water. Drain well and toss with the sesame oil. Set aside to cool completely.
3. Blanch the snow peas in boiling water until bright green and just tender. Refresh under cold running water and drain well.
4. Place the cooked noodles, snow peas, tofu, cucumber, ginger, spinach and cilantro in a large bowl. Pour over dressing and toss gently to combine. Divide the salad among 4 plates, top with the avocado, spring onions and cashews, and serve.

481 Cal, 26 g fat (saturated 5 g),
6 g fiber, 18 g protein, 41 g carbohydrate

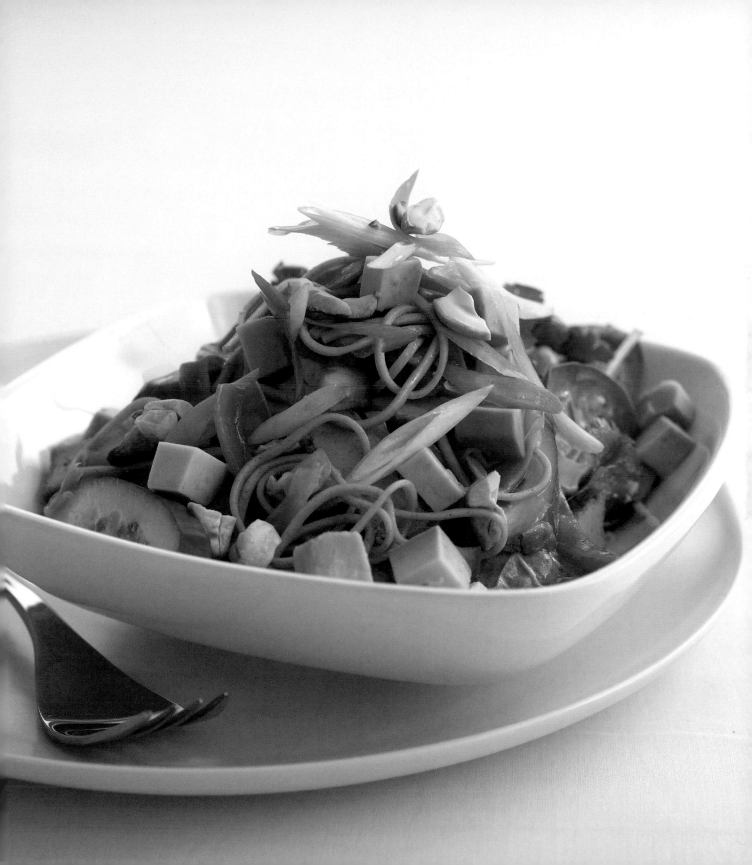

chickpea and red-kidney bean patties with avocado and corn salsa

Serves 4   Preparation time: 20 minutes   Cooking time: 10 minutes

1½ cups cooked red kidney beans
1⅓ cups cups cooked chickpeas
4 scallions, sliced
1 clove garlic
1 egg
⅓ cup couscous
salt and freshly ground black pepper
2 tablespoons olive oil
dressed salad leaves, to serve

AVOCADO AND CORN SALSA
1 cob corn
2 ripe tomatoes, finely chopped
1 small ripe avocado, finely chopped
½ small red onion, finely chopped
1 small red chile, finely chopped
⅓ cup finely chopped cilantro
2 tablespoons fresh lime juice
1 tablespoon olive oil
salt and freshly ground black pepper

1. To make the patties, place the kidney beans, chickpeas, spring onions, garlic and egg in a food processor. Process, occasionally scraping down the side of the bowl, until well combined. Transfer to a bowl. Stir in the couscous, season well, and set aside for 10 minutes. Using wet hands, shape the mixture into 8 patties. Refrigerate until required.
2. To make the Avocado and Corn Salsa, microwave or steam the corn until just tender. Set aside to cool slightly. Cut the kernels off the cob and place in a bowl with the tomato, avocado, onion, chile, cilantro, lime juice and oil. Stir gently, and season.
3. Heat the oil in a large, non-stick frying pan over medium heat. Add the patties and cook for 2–3 minutes each side, or until golden brown. (Cook in batches if necessary.)
4. Serve the patties with the salsa and dressed salad leaves on the side.

505 Cal, 31 g fat (saturated 6 g),
12 g fiber, 17 g protein, 34 g carbohydrate

ricotta, feta and spinach filo triangles

Makes 12 Preparation time: 10 minutes Cooking time: 25–30 minutes

9 oz package frozen spinach, thawed
5½ oz low fat ricotta
3½ oz low fat feta, crumbled
¼ cup chopped flat-leaf parsley
2 scallions, finely chopped
pinch nutmeg
salt and freshly ground black pepper
12 sheets filo pastry
1 tablespoon olive oil

1. Preheat oven to 350°F. Line two baking trays with parchment paper.
2. Squeeze all the excess moisture out of the spinach. Place the ricotta and feta in a bowl and use a fork to combine them. Add the spinach, parsley, scallion and nutmeg. Mix until well combined and season well.
3. Place one sheet of pastry on a clean surface. Fold over lengthways. Place one-twelfth of the spinach mixture in one corner of the pastry. Fold pastry over to form a triangle and continue folding to the end of the pastry. Place on one of the trays and brush the top with oil. Repeat with the remaining pastry and spinach mixture.
4. Bake the triangles for 25–30 minutes, or until golden brown.

96 Cal, 4 g fat (saturated 2 g),
2 g fiber, 6 g protein, 8 g carbohydrate

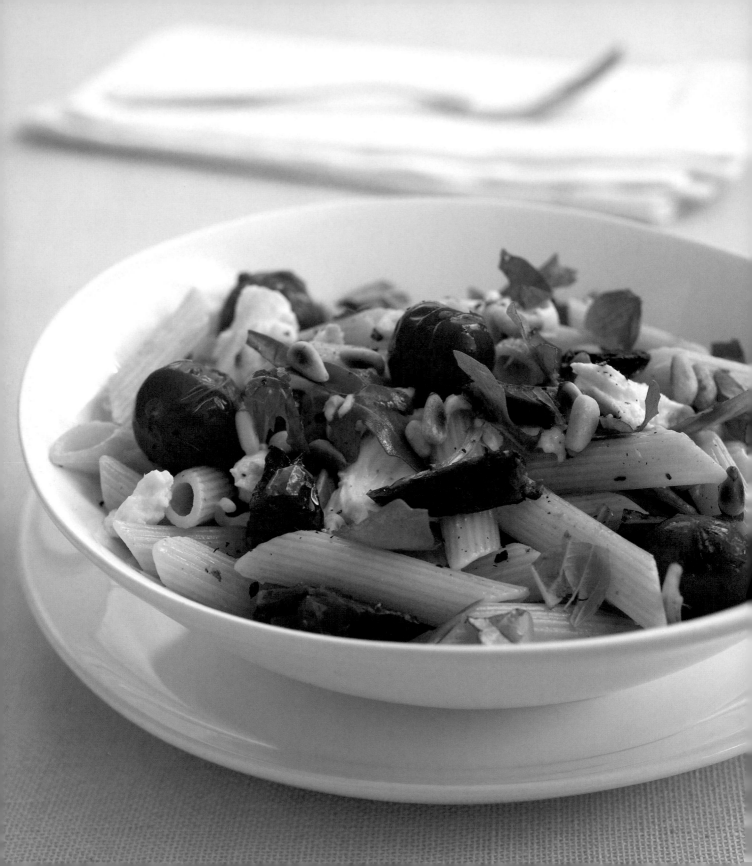

main dishes

These recipes are more substantial options for the main meal of the day.
Packed with flavor and bursting with micronutrients, they include
a healthy balance of protein, carbohydrates and the right fats to give your
body the fuel it requires. We've included a wide variety of foods and
cooking methods to show you how easy and delicious using fresh, simple,
unprocessed ingredients (and lots of low GI carbs) can be.

penne with tomatoes, buffalo mozzarella and fresh basil

Serves 4 Preparation time: 10 minutes Cooking time: 15 minutes (*pictured on page 120*)

11¼ oz dried penne
1 tablespoon olive oil
1 clove garlic, crushed
5 oz or about 16 semi-dried tomatoes
9 oz small cherry tomatoes, roughly chopped
3½ oz buffalo mozzarella, torn into ¾ in pieces
1½ cups baby arugula, roughly chopped
⅓ cup picked basil leaves, torn
1 teaspoon finely grated lemon zest
freshly ground black pepper
¼ cup pine nuts, lightly toasted, to serve

If you are unable to find buffalo mozzarella, substitute with bocconcini or fresh mozzarella.

1. Cook the penne in a large saucepan of lightly salted boiling water according to packet directions, or until al dente. Drain, and keep warm.
2. Return the pan to a medium–low heat, add the oil and garlic, and cook, stirring, for 30 seconds. Add the semi-dried tomatoes and cherry tomatoes, increase the heat to medium–high and cook, stirring, for 2–3 minutes, or until the cherry tomatoes are slightly wilted. Add the drained penne and mix it well with the tomatoes and garlic.
3. Remove the pan from the heat, add the mozzarella, arugula, basil and lemon zest, and season with pepper.
4. Divide among 4 serving bowls and garnish with the pine nuts.

512 Cal, 20 g fat (saturated 5 g),
7 g fiber, 19 g protein, 61 g carbohydrate

butternut squash, spinach and ricotta manicotti

Serves 4 Preparation time: 25 minutes Cooking time: 1 hour Cooling time: 5 minutes

1 lb 2 oz butternut squash
 (14 oz peeled weight), peeled,
 cut into 1¼ in cubes
olive oil spray
2 teaspoons olive oil
1 small onion, finely chopped
1 clove garlic, crushed
14 oz low fat ricotta
13 oz package frozen spinach,
 thawed, squeezed of excess water
pinch nutmeg
salt and freshly ground black pepper
4 (12 x 6½ in) fresh lasagna sheets,
 cut in half crosswise
¼ cup finely grated parmesan

TOMATO SAUCE
2 teaspoons olive oil
1 onion, finely chopped
2 cloves garlic, crushed
1 teaspoon chopped thyme leaves
2 – 14 oz cans chopped tomatoes
pinch salt
pinch Superfine sugar
2 tablespoons chopped basil
freshly ground black pepper

1. To make the Tomato Sauce, heat the oil in a large heavy-based saucepan, add the onion and cook over medium–low heat, stirring occasionally, for 5–6 minutes, or until soft. Add the garlic and thyme and cook, stirring, for 1 minute more. Add the tomatoes, salt and sugar and simmer, stirring occasionally, for 20 minutes, or until slightly thick. Remove from heat, mix in the basil and season. Set aside.
2. Preheat oven to 350°F. Line a baking tray with baking paper.
3. Place the squash on the prepared tray and spray lightly with olive oil. Roast for 25 minutes, or until soft and lightly golden. Remove and set aside to cool a little.
4. Meanwhile, heat the olive oil in a small frying pan, add the onion and cook over medium–low heat for 5 minutes, or until soft. Add the garlic and cook, stirring, for 1 minute more.
5. Put the squash and the onion mixture together in a bowl. Add the ricotta, spinach and nutmeg. Use a fork to mash all ingredients together until well combined, then season.
6. Spread 4 tablespoons of the Tomato Sauce in the base of a 6 cup ovenproof baking dish. Place one cup of the squash filling down the middle of each lasagna sheet, then roll each lasagna sheet over to enclose the filling and make a tube shape. Place in dish. Cover with the remaining Tomato Sauce and top with the parmesan.
7. Bake for 25 minutes, or until bubbling. Set aside for 5 minutes before serving.

586 Cal, 18 g fat (saturated 8 g),
12 g fiber, 30 g protein, 73 g carbohydrate

spiralli with broccoli and pesto balsamico

Serves 4   Preparation time: 10 minutes   Cooking time: 15 minutes

11¼ oz spiralli (or other short pasta,
 such as fusilli, farfalle, penne)
10½ oz broccoli, cut into small florets
1 cup low fat ricotta
3 tablespoons good-quality basil pesto
1 tablespoon balsamic vinegar
2 tablespoons pine nuts, lightly toasted
1 cup baby spinach leaves, washed,
 shredded
¼ cup finely grated pecorino, to serve
freshly ground black pepper, to serve

This pasta is quick to make and delicious. You can substitute the broccoli with cauliflower florets, or try using arugula pesto instead of basil pesto.

1. Cook the pasta in a large saucepan of lightly salted boiling water according to package instructions, or until al dente.
2. Meanwhile, steam the broccoli until bright green and just tender, and set aside. Place the ricotta and pesto in a small bowl and stir until well combined.
3. When the pasta is cooked, reserve ½ cup of the cooking liquid before draining well and returning the pasta to the pan. Add the balsamic vinegar to the pasta and toss, then add the ricotta mixture, pine nuts, spinach, broccoli and ¼ cup of the reserved cooking liquid. (Add a little more liquid, if necessary, to reach coating consistency.)
4. Serve immediately, sprinkled with the pecorino and pepper.

504 Cal, 19 g fat (saturated 6 g),
7 g fiber, 23 g protein, 60 g carbohydrate

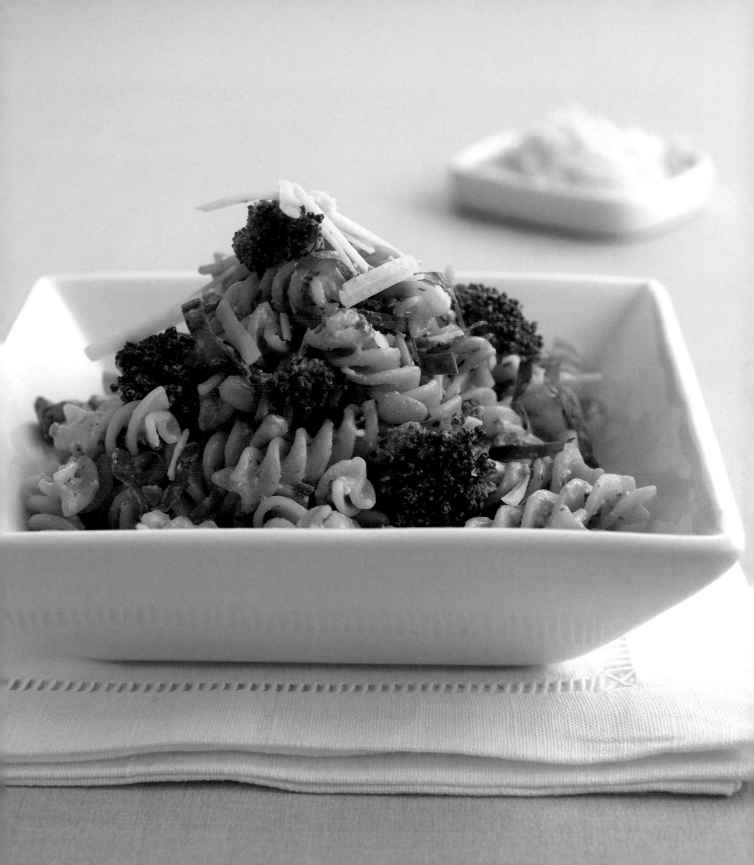

spaghetti with steamed greens and cranberry beans

Serves 4 Preparation time: 10 minutes Cooking time: 18 minutes

11¼ oz whole wheat (or regular)
  spaghetti
2 large zucchini, trimmed, cut into
  matchsticks
5½ oz snow peas, strings removed
1 bunch broccolini, trimmed and cut
  into long florets
1 bunch (5½ oz) asparagus, trimmed
  and cut into (around 1¼ in) lengths
1 teaspoon olive oil
1 – 14 oz can cranberry beans, rinsed
  and drained
8 basil leaves, torn
1 tablespoon sesame seeds,
  lightly toasted

DRESSING
1 tablespoon lemon juice
1 teaspoon finely grated lemon zest
2 tablespoons olive oil
1 clove garlic, crushed
salt and freshly ground black pepper
2 teaspoons sesame oil

You can use any combination of steamed greens in this recipe, such as peas, baby spinach and green beans.

1. To make the dressing, place all dressing ingredients in a small bowl and whisk to combine. Set aside.
2. Cook the spaghetti in a large saucepan of lightly salted boiling water according to package directions, or until al dente. Drain and keep warm.
3. Meanwhile, steam the zucchini, snow peas, broccolini and asparagus until bright green and just tender.
4. Return the pasta saucepan to the heat with the olive oil. Add the cranberry beans and gently heat. Return the pasta to the pan along with the steamed greens, and add the dressing and basil leaves. Sprinkle with the sesame seeds, and serve.

592 Cal 17 g fat (saturated 2 g),
7 g fiber, 25 g protein, 79 g carbohydrate

lentil, mushroom and ricotta lasagna

Serves 6 Preparation time: 20 minutes Cooking time: 1 hour Cooling time: 5 minutes

1 tablespoon olive oil

1 brown onion, finely chopped

1 carrot, peeled, finely chopped

1 stick celery, finely chopped

1 clove garlic, crushed

1 teaspoon freshly chopped thyme
  leaves

1 tablespoon tomato paste

1 – 14 oz can chopped tomatoes

1 – 14 oz can brown lentils, rinsed
  and drained

14 oz button mushrooms, sliced

salt and freshly ground black pepper

1 lb 2 oz low fat ricotta

1 egg

½ cup skim milk

pinch nutmeg

4 (12 x 6½ in) fresh lasagna sheets

¼ cup finely grated parmesan

1. Heat half the oil in a large, heavy-based saucepan over medium–low heat. Add the onion, carrot and celery and cook, stirring occasionally, for 6–8 minutes, or until the vegetables soften. Add the garlic and thyme and cook, stirring, for 1 minute. Add the tomato paste and cook, stirring, for 2 minutes. Add the tomatoes and lentils and cook, stirring occasionally, for 10 minutes, or until sauce thickens. Remove from heat and set aside.

2. Heat the remaining oil in a large pan, add the mushrooms and cook, stirring, for 3–4 minutes, or until slightly soft. Season and remove from heat.

3. Preheat oven to 350°F. Lightly oil an 8 cup ovenproof dish. Combine the ricotta, egg, milk and nutmeg in a bowl.

5. To assemble the lasagna, place a sheet of lasagna in the base of the prepared dish. Top with a third of the lentil mixture, scatter over a third of the mushrooms and smooth over a third of the ricotta mixture. Repeat these steps. Then top with a third lasagna sheet, the remaining lentils and mushrooms, then a fourth lasagna sheet, and finally the remaining ricotta. Sprinkle over the parmesan.

6. Bake for 30 minutes, or until top is golden and bubbling. Set aside to rest for 5 minutes before cutting.

429 Cal, 14 g fat (saturated 6 g),
7 g fiber, 24 g protein, 50 g carbohydrate

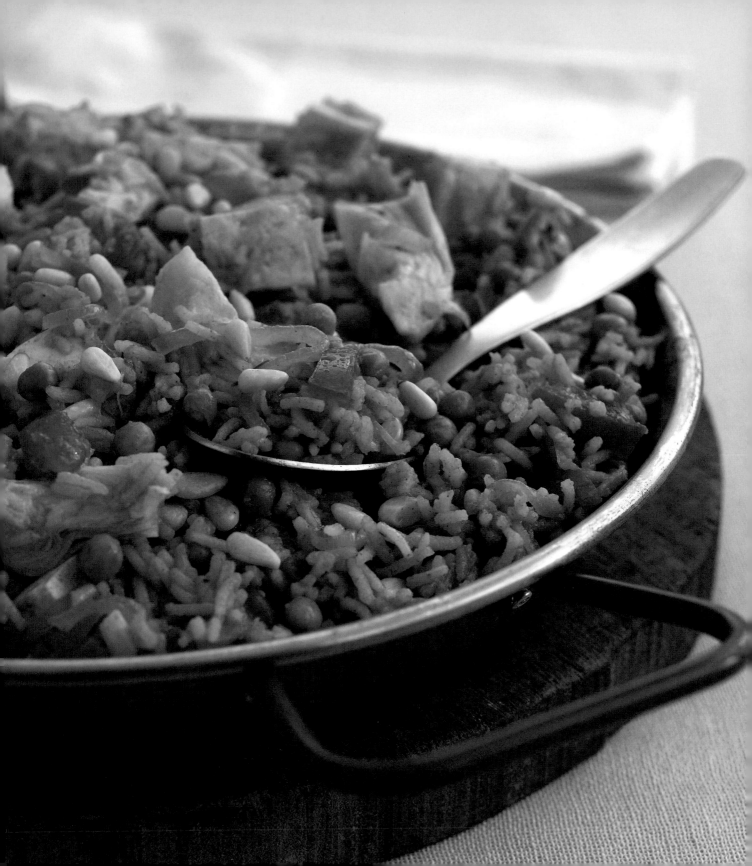

vegetarian paella

Serves 6–8   Preparation time: 20 minutes   Cooking time: 35 minutes

1 tablespoon olive oil

2 red onions, thinly sliced

2 cloves garlic, crushed

1 teaspoon sweet smoked paprika

2 teaspoons paprika

10½ oz basmati rice

½ teaspoon saffron strands

4 cups good-quality vegetable stock

1 red pepper, roasted, peeled, sliced

1 green pepper, roasted, peeled, sliced

2 vine-ripened tomatoes, deseeded, chopped

¾ cup fresh corn kernels (about 1 large cob)

1 cup frozen baby peas, thawed

10½ oz firm tofu, cut into ¾ in chunks

6 oz drained marinated artichoke hearts, cut into thin wedges

⅓ cup pine nuts, lightly toasted, to serve

Paella makes a fantastic addition to a party menu. It is easy to prepare, as it is all cooked in the one pan. You can add practically anything you like.

1. Heat the oil in a large, heavy-based saucepan over medium–low heat. Add the onion and cook, stirring occasionally, for 5–6 minutes, or until onion is soft. Add the garlic and cook, stirring, for 1 minute. Add the paprikas and cook, stirring, for 1 minute more. Add the rice and stir to coat the grains in the spices.

2. Add the saffron to the vegetable stock, then add the stock to the rice. Bring to the boil, then reduce heat to low, cover the pan with a lid or piece of foil and simmer for 20–25 minutes, or until the stock is absorbed and the rice is cooked.

3. Add the peppers, tomato, corn, peas and tofu, stir to combine, cover again and cook for a further 5 minutes. Remove from the heat and mix in the artichokes. Serve garnished with the pine nuts.

361 Cal, 12 g fat (saturated 2 g),
6 g fiber, 15 g protein, 45 g carbohydrate

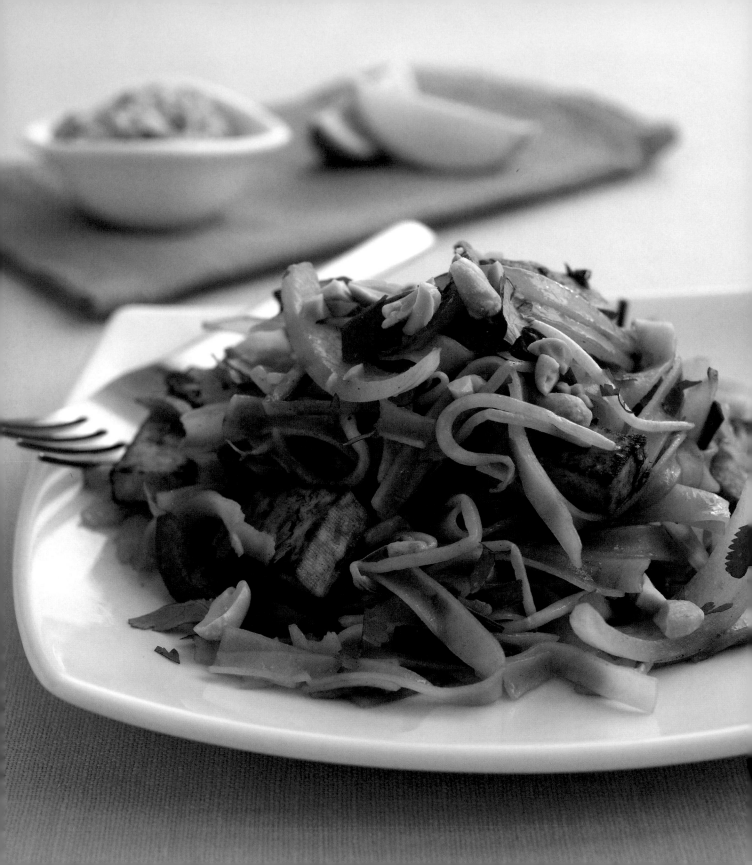

vegetarian pad thai

Serves 4 Preparation time: 15 minutes Marinating time: 30 minutes Cooking time: 15 minutes

10½ oz firm tofu, cut into cubes

¼ cup light soy sauce

1 tablespoon kecap manis

1 clove garlic, crushed

2 teaspoons finely grated ginger

2 tablespoons lime juice

1 teaspoon Superfine sugar

7 oz dried flat rice noodles

1 tablespoon vegetable oil (such as canola)

1 brown onion, cut into thin wedges

1 long red chile, deseeded, cut into thin strips

1 red pepper, halved, deseeded, thinly sliced

1¼ cups bean sprouts, trimmed

¼ cup chopped garlic chives

2 tablespoons freshly chopped cilantro

¼ cup crushed unsalted peanuts, to serve

lime wedges, to serve

1. Place the tofu in a shallow, non-metallic dish. Combine 2 tablespoons of the soy sauce, the kecap manis, garlic and the ginger. Pour over the tofu, cover and set aside to marinate for at least 30 minutes.

2. Place the remaining soy sauce, lime juice and sugar in a small bowl. Set aside.

3. Place the noodles in a heatproof bowl, add enough boiling water to cover, and stand for 5 minutes. Drain and set aside.

4. Heat half the oil in a wok over high heat. With a slotted spoon add the tofu in batches and cook for 2–3 minutes, or until golden brown. Remove from wok and set aside.

5. Add remaining oil to wok with onion and chile and stir-fry for 2 minutes. Add the pepper and bean sprouts and stir-fry for 1 minute more.

6. Add the reserved noodles, lime juice mixture, garlic chives and cilantro to the wok and toss gently over high heat for 2 minutes, or until noodles are coated in the sauce and heated through. Return the tofu to the wok and cook for 1 minute more.

7. Serve immediately, sprinkled with the peanuts and accompanied by lime wedges.

374 Cal, 15 g fat (saturated 2 g),
5 g fiber, 18 g protein, 39 g carbohydrate

vegetarian shepherd's pie

Serves 4 Preparation time: 20 minutes Cooking time: 35 minutes

2 medium potatoes (about 10½ oz
  each), peeled, cut into chunks
1 small orange sweet potato (about
  10½ oz) peeled, cut into chunks
2 teaspoons mustard seed oil
salt and freshly ground black pepper
1 tablespoon olive oil
1 onion, finely chopped
1 carrot, peeled, finely chopped
1 stick celery, finely chopped
1 medium zucchini, finely chopped
4 oz button mushrooms, sliced
2 cloves garlic, crushed
2 tablespoons tomato paste
1 – 14 oz can lentils, rinsed and
  drained
1 – 14 oz can chopped tomatoes
1 tablespoon freshly chopped flat-leaf
  parsley
¼ cup grated low fat cheddar cheese
  (optional)
¼ cup fresh sourdough bread crumbs

If you are unable to find mustard seed oil, you can substitute it with olive oil or low fat margarine.

1. Boil the potato and sweet potato together in a medium-sized saucepan for 15 minutes, or until soft. Drain, add the mustard seed oil, season and mash until smooth.
2. Meanwhile, heat the olive oil in a large, heavy-based saucepan over medium–low heat. Add the onion, carrot and celery and cook, stirring occasionally, for 6–7 minutes, or until vegetables are slightly soft. Add the zucchini, mushrooms and garlic, and cook, stirring occasionally, for 3–4 minutes more. Add the tomato paste and cook, stirring, for 2 minutes. Add the lentils, tomatoes and ¼ cup water, and stir to combine. Simmer, stirring occasionally, for 10 minutes. mix in the chopped parsley.
3. Preheat the grill to high.
4. Spoon lentil mixture into a 6 cup ovenproof dish. Top with the mashed potato mix and sprinkle with grated cheese, if using, and bread crumbs. Grill for 5–10 minutes, or until top is golden and bubbling. Serve immediately.

295 Cal, 8 g fat (saturated 1 g),
9 g fiber, 4 g protein, 36 g carbohydrate

stuffed vegetables

Serves 4 Preparation time: 25 minutes Cooking time: 1 hour

½ cup pearl barley
⅓ cup quinoa
2 medium-sized eggplants, halved lengthwise
6 large vine-ripened tomatoes
1 tablespoon olive oil
1 onion, finely chopped
1 stick celery, chopped
2 cloves garlic, crushed
2 teaspoons ground cumin
1 teaspoon dried oregano
1 zucchini, finely chopped
¼ cup pine nuts
¼ cup pumpkin seeds
2 tablespoons freshly chopped mint
2 tablespoons freshly chopped parsley
finely grated zest of 1 lemon
salt and freshly ground black pepper
2 red peppers, halved lengthways, deseeded

You could substitute the pearl barley and quinoa with cooked brown rice or couscous. Any variety of fresh herbs, vegetables, nuts and seeds can be added to the stuffing mix.

1. Place the pearl barley, quinoa and 3 cups water in a medium-sized saucepan. Bring to the boil, then cover and simmer for 30 minutes, or until grains are tender. Drain well.
2. Meanwhile, scoop out the flesh of the eggplants, leaving a ½ in thick shell. Sprinkle the insides with salt and place upside down on a paper towel to drain off the bitter juices. Dice the flesh.
3. Preheat oven to 350°F. Deseed and dice 2 of the tomatoes. Cut the tops off the remaining 4 tomatoes and scoop out their seeds, leaving a shell. Set aside.
4. Heat the oil in a large frying pan over medium–low heat. Add the onion and celery and cook, stirring occasionally, for 5 minutes, or until vegetables are soft. Add the garlic, cumin, oregano and zucchini and cook, stirring, for 1 minute. Increase the heat to medium–high, add the chopped eggplant and zucchini and cook, stirring, for 2–3 minutes, or until lightly golden. Add the drained barley and quinoa, the chopped tomato, pine nuts, pumpkin seeds, mint, parsley and lemon zest, and season.
5. Rinse out the eggplant shells and pat dry. Fill the eggplants, tomatoes and peppers with the stuffing mixture, place on a lightly oiled baking tray and roast for 30 minutes, or until vegetables are soft and golden brown. Serve.

368 Cal, 19 g fat (saturated 2 g),
13 g fiber, 12 g protein, 31 g carbohydrate

brown rice and barley salad with spiced chickpeas, sweet potato and currants

Serves 4 Preparation time: 20 minutes Cooking time: 25 minutes

⅔ cup brown rice

¾ cup pearl barley

3 teaspoons ground cumin

1 small (around 9 oz) sweet potato, peeled, cut into ¾ in pieces

1 red onion, cut into thin wedges

1 – 14 oz can chickpeas, rinsed, drained

1 teaspoon ground cilantro

1 teaspoon paprika

½ teaspoon turmeric

1 tablespoon olive oil

⅓ cup currants

⅓ cup lightly toasted slivered almonds

2 tablespoons freshly chopped cilantro

3 cups arugula leaves

salt and freshly ground black pepper

Yogurt Tahini Dressing (see recipe page 174), to serve

By combining brown rice with barley, you lower the overall GI of the meal. Adding spices and roasting the chickpeas is a great way to add lots of flavour. Low fat yogurt is fantastic for creating healthy, creamy dressings.

1. Preheat oven to 350°F. Line a baking tray with baking paper.

2. Cook the brown rice and pearl barley in two separate large saucepans of boiling water, with one teaspoon of cumin added to each pan. Cook, stirring occasionally, for 25 minutes, or until al dente (the pearl barley will take a little longer). Drain well.

3. Meanwhile, place the sweet potato, onion and chickpeas in a large bowl. Mix the remaining cumin, ground cilantro, paprika, turmeric and the oil together, then add to the bowl with the sweet potato mixture and toss to coat evenly. Place the mixture in a single layer on the prepared baking tray and bake for 20 minutes, or until the sweet potato is just tender.

4. Toss the rice, barley, sweet potato mixture, currants, almonds, chopped cilantro, arugula leaves together in a large bowl. Season and serve drizzled with a little Yogurt Tahini Dressing.

602 Cal, 16 g fat (saturated 2 g), 14 g fiber, 20 g protein, 87 g carbohydrate

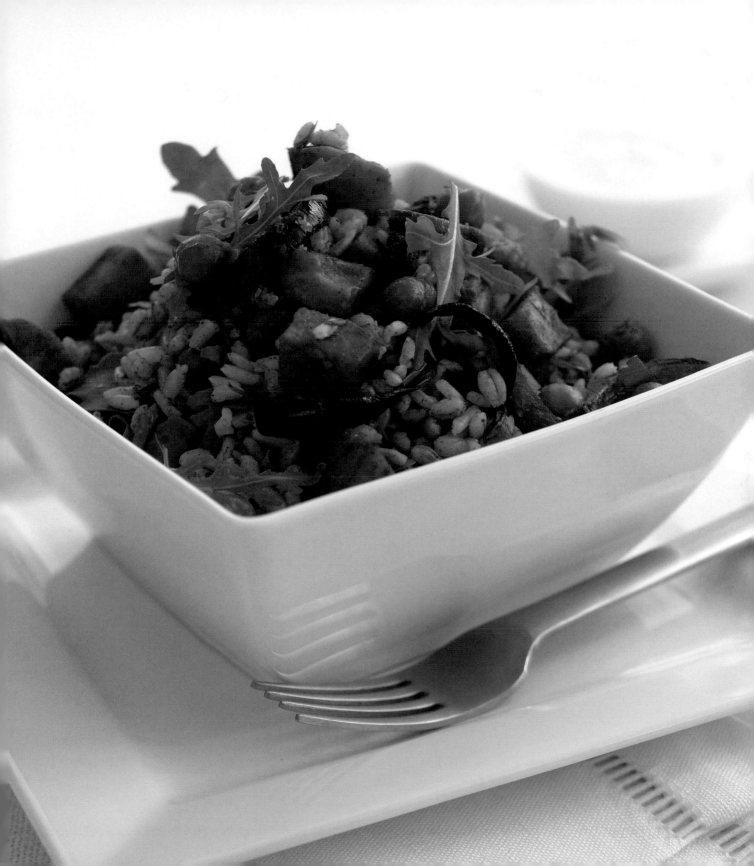

three-bean chili with spicy tortilla crisps

Serves 4   Preparation time: 20 minutes   Soaking time: overnight   Cooking time: 50 minutes

1 tablespoon olive oil

1 brown onion, finely chopped

1 carrot, peeled, finely chopped

1 stick celery, finely chopped

2 cloves garlic, crushed

1 long red chile, finely chopped

½ teaspoon chili powder

½ teaspoon dried oregano

1 small red pepper, deseeded, finely
  chopped

1 small green pepper, deseeded, finely
  chopped

2 small zucchini, sliced

2 tablespoons tomato paste

1 – 14 oz can chopped tomatoes

1 cup vegetable stock

½ cup bulgur (cracked wheat)

1 – 14 oz can red kidney beans,
  rinsed and drained

½ cup black-eyed beans, soaked
  overnight

salt and freshly ground black pepper

juice of 1 lime

2 tablespoons chopped cilantro

SPICY TORTILLA CRISPS

4 purchased corn tortillas

olive oil spray

½ teaspoon paprika

¼ teaspoon chili powder

Guacamole goes particularly well with this recipe.

1. Heat the oil in a large heavy-based saucepan over medium–low heat. Add the onion, carrot and celery and cook, stirring occasionally, for 6–7 minutes, or until vegetables are slightly soft. Add the garlic, chile, chili powder and oregano and cook, stirring, for 1–2 minutes, or until fragrant. Add the pepper and zucchini and cook for 1 minute more.

2. Add the tomato paste and cook, stirring, for 1 minute. Add the chopped tomatoes and stock, and stir to combine. Add the bulgur and beans. Bring to the boil, then reduce the heat to very low and simmer, covered, stirring frequently, for 30 minutes, or until beans and vegetables are tender.

3. Season, add lime juice to taste, and mix in the chopped cilantro.

4. To make the Spicy Tortilla Crisps, preheat oven to 350°F. Spray both sides of each tortilla lightly with olive oil. Sprinkle with the paprika and chili powder. Place the tortillas on a large baking tray and bake in the oven for 5–6 minutes, or until crisp. Cut into quarters and serve with the Three-Bean Chili.

COOK'S TIP

You can use any spices on these tortillas, such as ground cilantro, cumin or cayenne pepper.

296 Cal, 7 g fat (saturated 1 g),
14 g fiber, 14 g protein, 38 g carbohydrate

moroccan bean and pumpkin tagine

Serves 4 Preparation time: 20 minutes Cooking time: 20 minutes

1 tablespoon olive oil

1 onion, finely chopped

2 cloves garlic, crushed

2 teaspoons finely grated fresh ginger

4 teaspoons Herbie's Tagine Spice Mix
  (see recipe page 174)

1 lb 2 oz pumpkin, peeled, deseeded,
  cut into 1¼ in cubes

2 carrots, cut into bite-sized chunks

2 cups good-quality vegetable stock

5½ oz green beans, trimmed, cut into
  1½ in lengths

12 pitted prunes

2 teaspoons pure floral honey

14 oz can butter beans

salt and freshly ground black pepper

1 tablespoon freshly chopped cilantro

¼ cup sliced almonds, lightly toasted,
  to serve

Casablancan Couscous
  (see recipe page 174), to serve

This tagine uses butter beans, but you can use any type of canned bean or lentil.

1. Heat the oil in a large, heavy-based pan over medium—low heat. Add the onion and cook, stirring occasionally, for 5 minutes, or until soft. Add the garlic, ginger and Spice Mix and cook, stirring, for 1–2 minutes, or until fragrant. Add the pumpkin and carrots and cook for a further 1 minute.

2. Add the stock, bring to a boil then reduce the heat and simmer for 15 minutes, or until vegetables are tender. Add the green beans, prunes and honey. Simmer for a further 3–4 minutes, or until beans are just cooked. Add the butter beans and cook for a further 1 minute, or until heated through.

3. Season, mix in the cilantro and sprinkle with the sliced almonds. Serve with Casablancan Couscous.

610 Cal, 14 g fat (saturated 2 g)
7 g fiber, 19 g protein, 98 g carbohydrate

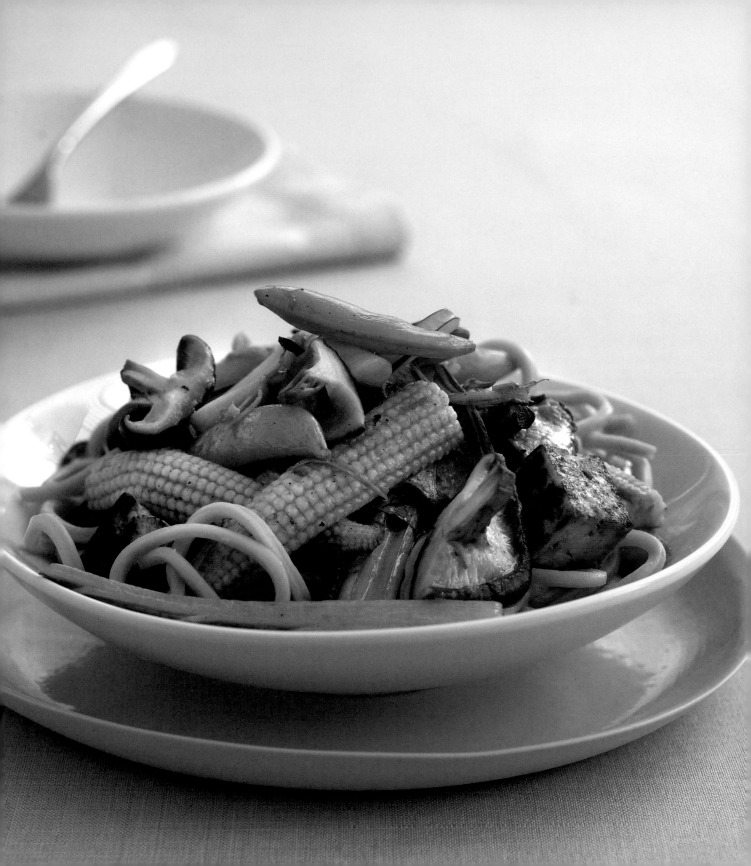

shiitake, ginger and tofu hokkien noodles

Serves 4 Preparation time: 15 minutes Marinating time: 4 hours Cooking time: 10 minutes

2 tablespoons soy sauce

2 tablespoons Chinese rice wine

1 tablespoon Chinese black vinegar

1 clove garlic, crushed

2 teaspoons finely grated ginger

1 – 13 oz packet firm tofu, cut into
⅝ in cubes

1 lb package hokkien noodles

1 tablespoon olive oil

1¼ in piece ginger, cut into very thin
matchsticks

1 long red chile, deseeded, thinly
sliced

5½ oz baby corn, halved lengthwise

5½ oz fresh shiitake mushrooms,
halved

5½ oz sugar snap peas, strings
removed

6 scallions, trimmed, cut into
1½ in lengths

1 bunch choy sum, trimmed, cut into
3 equal lengths

Chinese black vinegar is available from Asian supermarkets. It's a delicious addition to Asian stir-fries, marinades and salad dressings.

1. Combine the soy sauce, rice wine, vinegar, garlic and grated ginger in a shallow, non-metallic dish. Add the tofu and turn to coat in the marinade. Cover and refrigerate for 4 hours, turning once.

2. Meanwhile, place the noodles in a large heatproof bowl and cover with boiling water. Set aside for 5 minutes, then drain well.

3. Heat half the oil in a large wok or frying pan. With a slotted spoon add the tofu (reserving the marinade) in batches and fry until golden. Remove and set aside.

4. Heat the remaining oil, add the sliced ginger and chile and stir-fry for 30 seconds. Add the baby corn and mushrooms and stir-fry for 2 minutes more. Add the sugar snap peas and scallion and cook for 1 minute, then add the choy sum and reserved marinade. Toss together for 1–2 minutes over heat. Return the tofu to the wok and toss to combine and heat through.

5. Place the noodles in bowls and top with the vegetables and marinade liquid.

390 Cal, 12 g fat (saturated 2 g),
8 g fiber, 20 g protein, 44 g carbohydrate

grilled vegetable skewers with grilled corn

Serves 4   Preparation time: 15 minutes   Marinating time: 3–4 hours   Cooking time: 15 minutes

3 tablespoons soy sauce

2 tablespoons Chinese rice wine

2 teaspoons sesame oil

2 teaspoons freshly grated ginger

1 – 13 oz packet firm tofu, cut into
   ¾ in cubes

1 red pepper, deseeded, cut into ¾ in
   dice

1 yellow pepper, deseeded, cut into
   ¾ in dice

1 red onion, cut into ¾ in dice

1 zucchini, trimmed, cut into ¾ in
   chunks

16 cherry tomatoes

16 button mushrooms, trimmed

8 wooden skewers, soaked in cold
   water

vegetable oil, to brush

Barley and Red Rice Salad (see recipe
   page 177), to serve

GRILLED CORN

4 corn cobs, husks and silks removed

salt and freshly ground black pepper

1 lime, cut in half

1. To make the Grilled Corn, preheat a grill pan to high. Season each cob, squeeze over a little lime juice, then wrap each in aluminium foil. Grill, turning frequently, for 10 minutes, or until tender.

2. To make the Grilled Vegetable Skewers, mix together the soy sauce, rice wine, sesame oil and ginger in a shallow, non-metallic dish. Add the tofu and stir to coat in the marinade. Cover and refrigerate, turning once, for 3–4 hours.

3. Preheat a grill pan on high.

4. Thread the tofu, peppers, onion, zucchini, tomatoes and mushrooms on the skewers. Brush the skewers with the vegetable oil.

5. Cook the skewers, brushing occasionally with the remaining marinade, for 2–3 minutes each side, or until vegetables and tofu are cooked through and lightly charred. Serve with the Grilled Corn, and Barley and Red Rice Salad.

467 Cal, 13 g fat (saturated 2 g),
11 g fiber, 21 g protein, 59 g carbohydrate

lentil and vegetable nut roast

Makes 8 slices (serves 4) Preparation time: 20 minutes Cooking time: 1 hour Cooling time: 10 minutes

⅓ cup red lentils

½ cup green lentils

1½ cups good-quality vegetable stock

1 bay leaf

2 teaspoons olive oil

1 onion, finely chopped

1 stick celery, finely chopped

1 clove garlic, crushed

2 teaspoons ground cilantro

1 teaspoon ground cumin

4½ oz mushrooms, finely chopped

1 red pepper, deseeded, finely
  chopped

1½ cups loosely packed whole grain
  bread crumbs

½ cup hazelnut meal

2 eggs, lightly beaten

2 tablespoons chopped cilantro

zest and juice of ½ lemon

salt and freshly ground black pepper

⅓ cup hazelnuts, lightly toasted, skins
  removed, chopped

Chile Corn Salsa (see recipe page 175),
  to serve

1. Wash the lentils and place in a large saucepan with the stock and bay leaf. Bring to the boil, then reduce the heat and simmer for 20–30 minutes, or until the lentils are soft and the liquid is absorbed.

2. Meanwhile, preheat oven to 350°F. Line a 4 cup loaf tin with baking paper.

3. Heat the oil in a large saucepan over medium–low heat. Cook the onion and celery, stirring occasionally, for 5 minutes, or until they begin to soften. Add the garlic, ground cilantro and cumin and cook, stirring, for 1 minute, or until fragrant. Add the mushrooms and pepper and cook for a further 2 minutes.

4. Remove the bay leaf from the lentils and add the lentils to the pan containing the vegetables. Add the bread crumbs, hazelnut meal, eggs, chopped cilantro, lemon zest and juice. Season.

5. Spoon the mixture into the prepared loaf tin, sprinkle over the chopped hazelnuts and bake for 35–40 minutes, or until firm to the touch and golden brown. Remove from the oven and allow to cool in the tin for 10 minutes before turning out.

6. Serve hot or cold in thick slices with Chile Corn Salsa.

606 Cal, 28 g fat (saturated 3 g),
15 g fiber, 28 g protein, 54 g carbohydrate

vegetarian fried rice

Serves 4   Preparation time: 15 minutes   Cooking time: 25 minutes

1¼ cups brown long-grain rice

1 tablespoon olive oil

3 eggs, at room temperature

1 long red chile, deseeded, thinly
  sliced

1 garlic clove, crushed

2 teaspoons finely grated ginger

1 red pepper, deseeded, thinly sliced

1 fresh corn cob, kernels removed

½ Chinese cabbage, trimmed,
  shredded

1 cup frozen peas, thawed

¾ cup bean sprouts, trimmed

4 scallions, trimmed, thinly sliced

2 tablespoons light soy sauce

1 tablespoon kecap manis, plus extra
  to serve

⅓ cup cashews, lightly toasted,
  roughly chopped, to serve

1. Cook the rice in a large saucepan of boiling water for
25 minutes, or until tender. Drain well. Spread out in a single
layer over two baking trays and set aside to cool completely.
2. Meanwhile, heat half the oil in a large non-stick wok or
frying pan over medium heat. Whisk the eggs until frothy.
Pour into the wok and swirl to cover the base. Cook for
2 minutes, or until the egg is set. Carefully loosen the edges,
turn out onto a board and allow to cool. Roll up the omelet
and cut into thin strips. Set aside.
3. Heat the remaining oil in a wok over high heat. Add the
chile, garlic and ginger and stir-fry for 30 seconds. Add the
pepper, corn, cabbage and peas and cook, tossing, for
2 minutes. Add the cooled rice and toss until heated through.
Add the sliced omelet (reserving a few slices for garnishing),
the bean sprouts, scallions, soy sauce and kecap manis, and
toss to combine.
4. Transfer fried rice to a serving dish, and serve garnished
with the cashew nuts and reserved omelet slices, and drizzled
with a little extra kecap manis, if desired.

507 Cal, 18 g fat (saturated 3 g),
10 g fiber, 19 g protein, 63 g carbohydrate

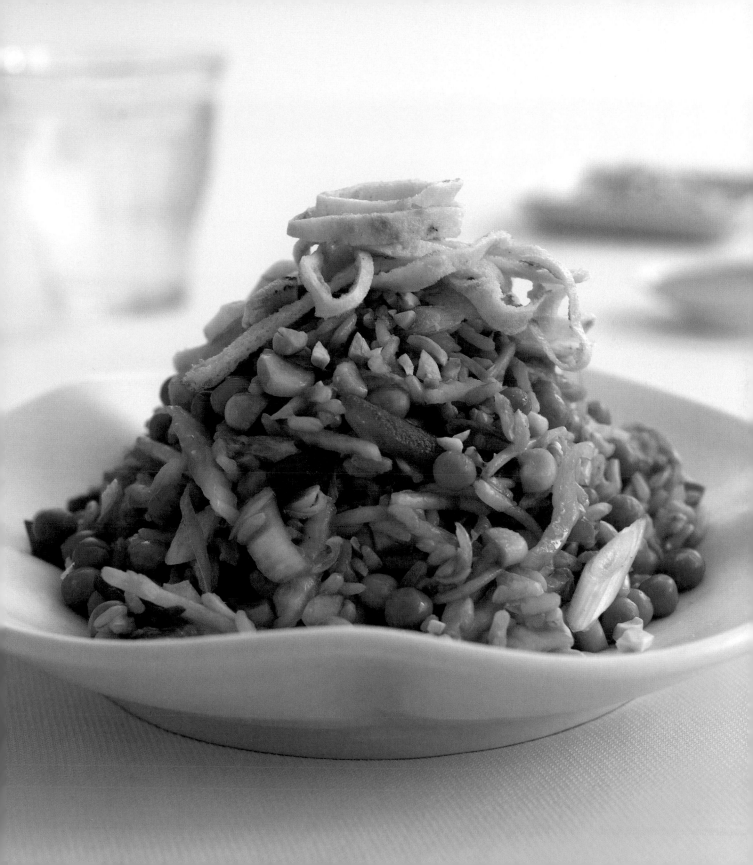

lentil and sunflower-seed burgers

Makes 4 Preparation time: 15 minutes Cooking time: 12 minutes Chilling time: 2–3 hours

1 – 14 oz can brown lentils, rinsed
  and drained
1½ tablespoons olive oil
1 small onion, finely chopped
1 clove garlic, crushed
1 carrot, finely chopped
⅓ cup sunflower seeds
½ cup rolled oats
½ cup whole grain bread crumbs
1 tablespoon soy sauce
whole wheat plain flour, to dust
4 whole wheat bread rolls, to serve
Tomato and Bean Salsa (see recipe
  page 175), to serve
baby arugula leaves, to serve

1. Place the lentils in a food processor and process until they resemble rough crumbs.
2. Heat ½ tablespoon of oil in a medium-sized frying pan, add the onion and cook, stirring, over medium–low heat for 5 minutes, or until soft. Add the garlic and cook, stirring, for 1 minute more. Add the carrot and cook, stirring, for a further 2 minutes.
3. Place the lentils, onion mixture, sunflower seeds, oats, bread crumbs and soy sauce in a large bowl and, using clean hands, mix to combine. Shape into 4 flat patties, then refrigerate for 2–3 hours, or until firm.
4. Dust each patty with flour. Heat the remaining olive oil in a large frying pan over medium–high heat. Add the patties and cook for 3–4 minutes each side, or until golden brown. Remove and drain on paper towels.
5. Assemble the burgers with the patties, rolls, Tomato and Bean Salsa and arugula, and serve.

592 Cal, 21 g fat (saturated 3 g),
9 g fiber, 23 g protein, 68 g carbohydrate

chickpea and vegetable curry with cumin-flavored rice

Serves 4   Preparation time: 15 minutes   Standing time: 30 minutes   Cooking time: 20 minutes

1 tablespoon canola oil

1 large onion, finely chopped

1 clove garlic, finely chopped

2 teaspoons finely grated ginger

2 teaspoons ground cilantro

1 teaspoon ground chili (or to taste)

1 teaspoon ground cumin

1 teaspoon garam masala

2 large vine-ripened tomatoes, chopped

1 – 14 oz can chickpeas, rinsed and
   drained

1 large carrot, peeled, chopped

1 small eggplant, trimmed, cut into
   ¾ in cubes

7 oz cauliflower, trimmed,
   cut into florets

2 teaspoons tamarind paste

1 teaspoon sugar

5½ oz green beans, trimmed, cut into
   1½ in lengths

salt and freshly ground black pepper
   (optional)

minted yogurt, to serve

CUMIN-FLAVORED RICE

1 cup basmati rice

1 teaspoon canola oil

2 teaspoons cumin seeds

This curry would also be delicious served with herbed couscous. It freezes well.

1. To cook the Cumin-flavored Rice, wash the rice well and place in a bowl, cover with cold water and soak for 30 minutes, then drain. Heat the oil in a heavy-based saucepan, add the cumin seeds and let them splutter until aromatic. Add the rice and 1½ cups water, stir and bring to the boil. Reduce the heat to very low, cover and cook for 15–20 minutes, or until all the water has evaporated.

2. Meanwhile, heat the oil in a heavy-based saucepan, add the onion and cook over medium–low heat for 5 minutes, or until soft. Add the garlic and ginger and cook, stirring, for 1 minute. Add the cilantro, chili, cumin and garam masala, and cook, stirring, for 1–2 minutes, or until aromatic. Add the tomato, chickpeas, carrot, eggplant, cauliflower and 1 cup water, bring to the boil, then reduce heat and stir in the tamarind paste and sugar. Simmer, partially covered, for 10 minutes, then add the beans and simmer for 5 minutes more. Season if desired.

3. Serve with Cumin-flavored Rice and minted yogurt.

405 Cal, 9 g fat (saturated 1 g),
11 g fiber, 14 g protein, 63 g carbohydrate

chickpea burgers

Serves 4   Preparation time: 20 minutes   Cooking time: 20 minutes   Chilling time: 2–3 hours

1 – 14 oz can chickpeas, rinsed and
  drained
1½ tablespoons olive oil
1 onion, finely chopped
1 clove garlic, crushed
1 tablespoon mild Indian curry paste
1 zucchini, grated
1½ cups firmly packed whole grain
  bread crumbs
1 tablespoon freshly chopped cilantro
¼ cup lightly toasted cashews,
  chopped
1 egg, lightly beaten
whole wheat all-purpose flour, to dust
4 whole grain bread rolls, to serve
Tomato and Bean Salsa (see recipe
  page 175), or fresh chopped tomato,
  to serve
sliced cucumber, to serve
baby arugula leaves, to serve

These burgers are delicious served with Tomato and Bean Salsa (see recipe page 175) or a purchased tomato salsa. You could also serve them as traditional burgers, with lettuce, beet and tomato.

1. Place the chickpeas in a food processor and process until they resemble fine crumbs.
2. Heat 2 teaspoons of the olive oil in a large frying pan over medium–low heat. Add the onion and cook, stirring occasionally, for 5 minutes, or until soft. Add the garlic and cook, stirring, for 1 minute. Add the curry paste and cook, stirring, for 1–2 minutes, or until fragrant. Add the zucchini and cook for 2 minutes more.
3. Transfer the onion mixture to a large bowl with the chickpeas, bread crumbs, cilantro, cashews and egg. Using clean hands, mix until all the ingredients are well combined, adding more bread crumbs if the mixture is too wet. Dust your hands with flour and shape the mixture into 4 flat patties. Refrigerate for 2–3 hours, or until firm.
4. Heat the remaining olive oil in a large frying pan over medium–high heat. Add the patties and cook for 3–4 minutes each side, or until golden. Remove and drain on paper towels.
5. Assemble the burgers with the patties, rolls, Tomato and Bean Salsa, cucumber slices and arugula, and serve.

623 Cal, 20 g fat (saturated 3 g),
20 g fiber, 25 g protein, 74 g carbohydrate

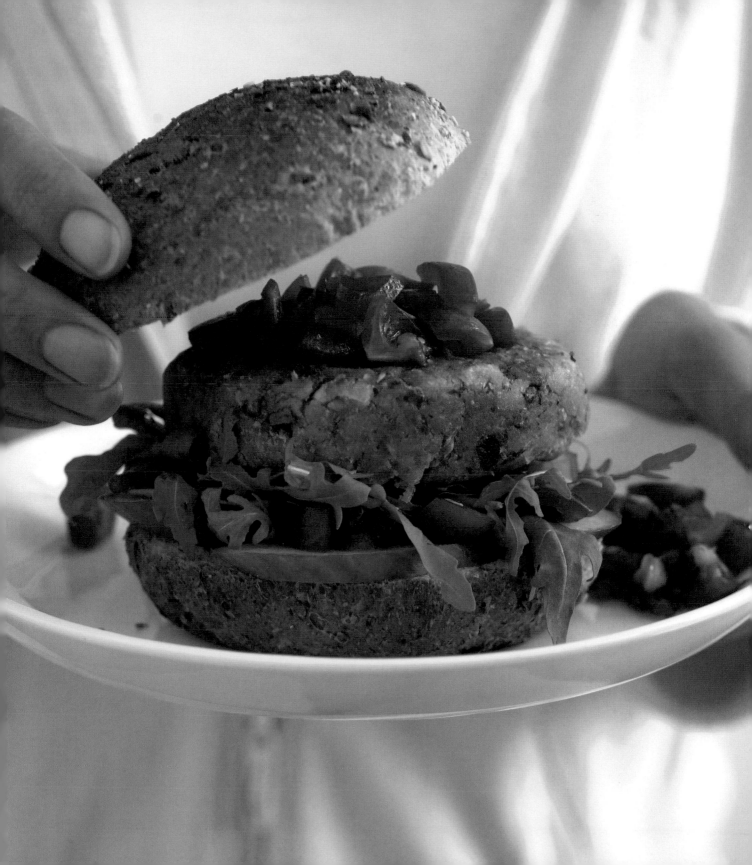

falafel rolls with hummus, tabbouleh and spicy tomato sauce

Serves 6

Preparation time: 60 minutes   Standing time: 20 minutes   Cooking time: 50 minutes

½ cup bulgur (cracked wheat)

2⅔ cups cooked chickpeas

1 onion, finely chopped

2 cloves garlic, crushed

2 teaspoons ground cilantro

1 teaspoon ground cumin

¼ teaspoon chili powder

⅓ cup firmly packed, picked flat-leaf parsley leaves

⅓ cup firmly packed picked cilantro leaves

salt and freshly ground black pepper

olive oil spray

Hummus (see recipe page 176)

6 rounds whole wheat pita bread

Tabbouleh (see recipe page 176)

Spicy Tomato Sauce (see recipe page 177)

The Hummus, Tabbouleh and Spicy Tomato Sauce (see pages 176 and 177) can be made ahead of time and stored in airtight containers in the fridge.

1. Place the bulgur in a small bowl and cover with ½ cup hot water. Set aside for 20 minutes, then place in a food processor with the chickpeas. Heat the oil in a small, non-stick frying pan over medium heat. Add the onion and garlic and cook, stirring, for 5–6 minutes, or until soft. Add the ground cilantro, cumin and chili powder and cook, stirring, for 1 minute. Add to the food processor along with the parsley and fresh cilantro, and process until well combined.

2. Preheat oven to 400°F. Line two baking trays with parchment paper.

3. Roll 1½ tablespoons of the falafel mixture into a ball, and flatten slightly. Repeat until you have used all the mixture. Place the falafels on the tray and spray the tops with oil. Cook for 25–30 minutes, or until slightly crisp on the outside and lightly golden.

4. Spread 2 tablespoons of Hummus over one side of each bread round. Top with ⅓ cup Tabbouleh, 3 falafels and 2 tablespoons Spicy Tomato Sauce. Roll up bread rounds, and serve.

599 Cal, 27 g fat (saturated 6 g), 17 g fiber, 20 g protein, 59 g carbohydrate

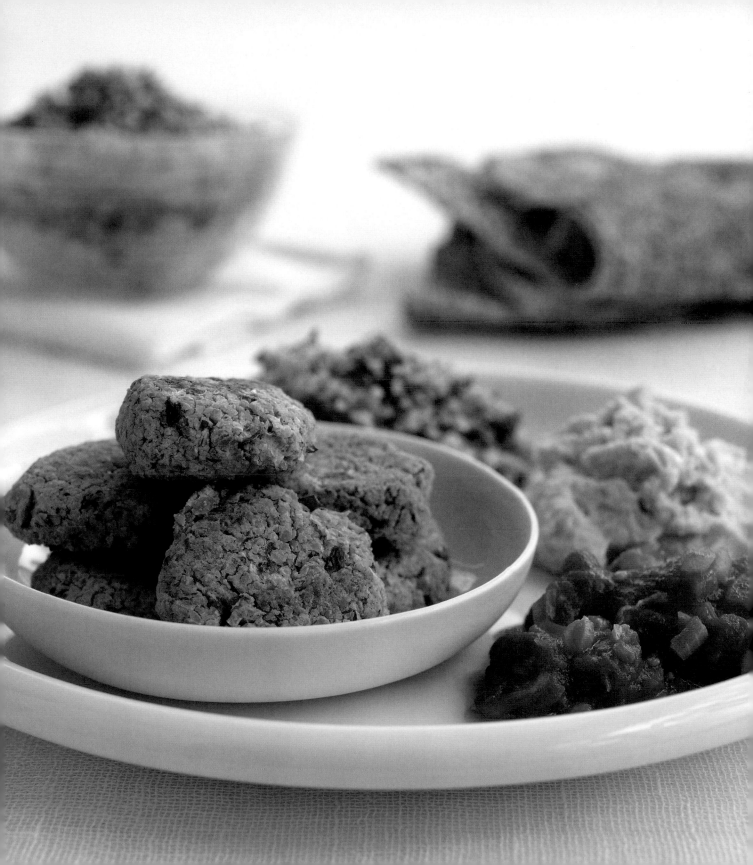

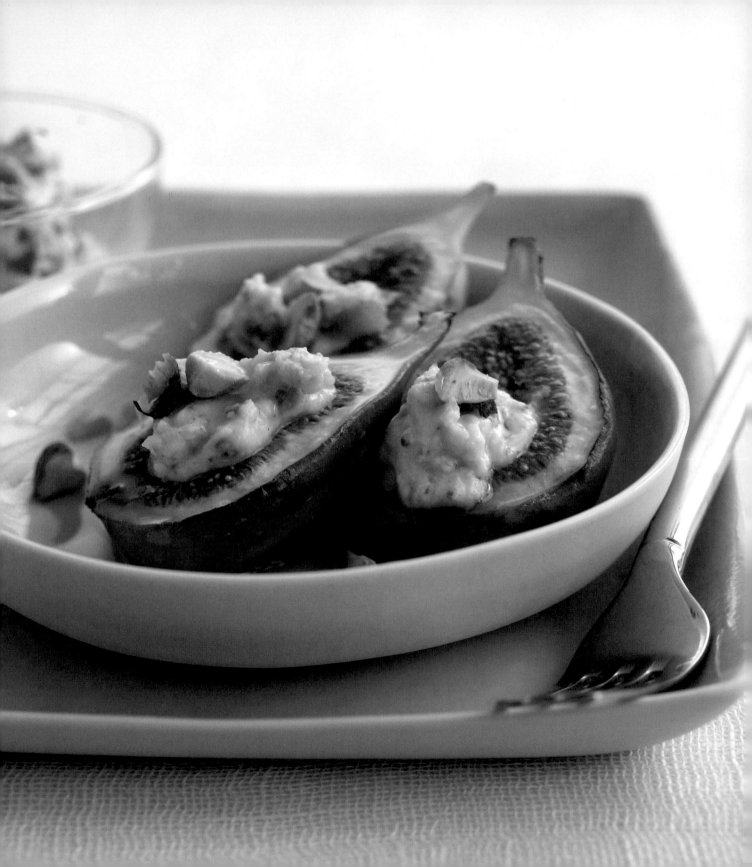

desserts and sweet snacks

If you center your desserts and sweet snacks around fruit and low fat dairy products, they can be a healthy low GI addition to your diet. The following recipes include traditional favorites and reinterpreted classics—plenty of inspiration, from dinner-party decadence to casual Sunday brunch, for every occasion.

honey-grilled figs with ricotta dolce

Serves 4   Preparation time: 10 minutes

Cooking time: 5 minutes (*pictured on page 150*)

4 large ripe figs
4 teaspoons pure floral honey or maple syrup
7 oz low fat ricotta
¼ cup carob buttons, finely chopped
1 oz glacé peaches, finely chopped
1 tablespoon powdered sugar, sifted
2 teaspoons amaretto
2 tablespoons chopped pistachios, plus extra,
   to garnish

1. Cut each fig in half and place on an ovenproof tray, cut side up. Drizzle half a teaspoon of honey over each fig.
2. Combine the ricotta, carob, glacé peach, powdered sugar, amaretto and pistachios in a medium-sized bowl, and stir until well combined.
3. Preheat grill to high. Grill figs for 2–3 minutes, or until slightly caramelized.
4. Divide among serving plates, top with a spoonful of the ricotta dolce, sprinkle with extra pistachios and serve immediately.

178 Cal, 8 g fat (saturated 5 g),
2 g fiber, 7 g protein, 20 g carbohydrate

star anise and lemongrass poached pears

Serves 4   Preparation time: 10 minutes

Cooking time: 30 minutes

5½ oz Superfine sugar
2 in piece ginger, peeled, thinly sliced
3 star anise
2 stems lemongrass, bruised, cut into 2 in lengths
2 strips lemon zest
4 medium-sized pears, peeled, cored and quartered
low fat yogurt, to serve

1. Place the sugar, ginger, star anise, lemongrass and lemon zest with 4 cups water in a large saucepan. Heat, stirring to dissolve the sugar. Bring to the boil, then reduce the heat to medium and simmer for 5 minutes.
2. Add the pears. Cover the top of the pears with a piece of baking paper and simmer for 15 minutes, or until tender. Remove pears with a slotted spoon and set aside. Continue to simmer the poaching liquid until reduced by half.
3. Serve the pears drizzled with the reduced liquid and a dollop of yogurt.

251 Cal, 0 g fat (saturated 0 g),
3 g fiber, 2 g protein, 60 g carbohydrate

summer berry pudding

Serves 4   Preparation time: 15 minutes   Cooking time: 5 minutes   Chilling time: overnight

1lb 2 oz fresh or frozen mixed berries,
  plus extra to serve
¼ cup raw sugar
1 cinnamon stick
8 slices sourdough bread, crusts
  removed
low fat yogurt or fromage frais,
  to serve

Frozen cherries, raspberries and blackberries are fantastic in this pudding—choose your own combination.

1. Combine the berries, sugar and cinnamon stick with ½ cup water in a medium-sized saucepan. Gently simmer for 5 minutes, or until the berries are plump and slightly soft. Discard the cinnamon stick and set the berries aside to cool.
2. Line a 2 cup soup bowl or mold with 6 slices of bread cut into triangles, overlapping to form a casing for the berries when the pudding is turned out. Cut the remaining 2 slices to fit the top of the bowl.
3. Spoon a little of the berry juice over the bread triangles to moisten, then, using a slotted spoon, fill the bowl with the berries. Pour around ½ cup of the berry juice over the berries and top with remaining bread slices to make a lid. Reserve any remaining berry juice.
4. Cover with plastic wrap and top with a plate to weigh down the pudding. Refrigerate overnight.
5. Turn the pudding out onto a white plate, and decorate with extra berries and any reserved juice, if desired. Serve with a dollop of yogurt.

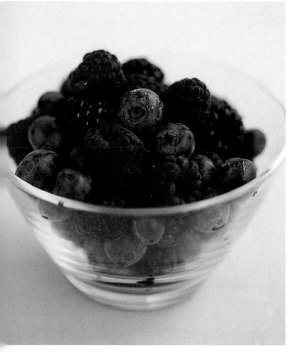

231 Cal, 2 g fat (saturated 0 g),
5 g fiber, 8 g protein, 44 g carbohydrate

poached peaches with vanilla yogurt and marinated raspberries

Serves 4   Preparation time: 10 minutes   Cooking time: 15 minutes   Cooling/chilling time: 2 hours

2 cups white wine
1 vanilla bean, split
½ cup Superfine sugar
4 large ripe freestone peaches
2 tablespoons fresh orange juice
2 teaspoons lime juice
1 tablespoon Superfine sugar, extra
1 cup fresh raspberries
low fat vanilla yogurt, to serve

1. Place the wine, vanilla bean and the sugar with 2 cups water in a saucepan and cook, stirring, over medium heat until the sugar dissolves. Simmer for 5 minutes.
2. Add the peaches and poach for a further 5 minutes. Remove the peaches with a slotted spoon, peel away their skins and set aside to cool to room temperature before placing in the refrigerator to chill.
3. Meanwhile, simmer the syrup until reduced by half. Strain into a bowl and allow to cool before placing in the refrigerator to chill.
4. Place the orange juice, lime juice and extra sugar in a medium-sized bowl, and stir to dissolve the sugar. Add the raspberries and toss to coat in the juice.
5. Serve the chilled peaches with the marinated raspberries, and drizzle with the chilled syrup. Accompany with a dollop of yogurt.

COOK'S TIP

You could substitute the peaches with nectarines in this recipe. Also, the fruit is still delicious when poached in water, as an alternative to water and wine.

313 Cal, 0 g fat (saturated 0 g),
5 g fiber, 4 g protein, 52 g carbohydrate

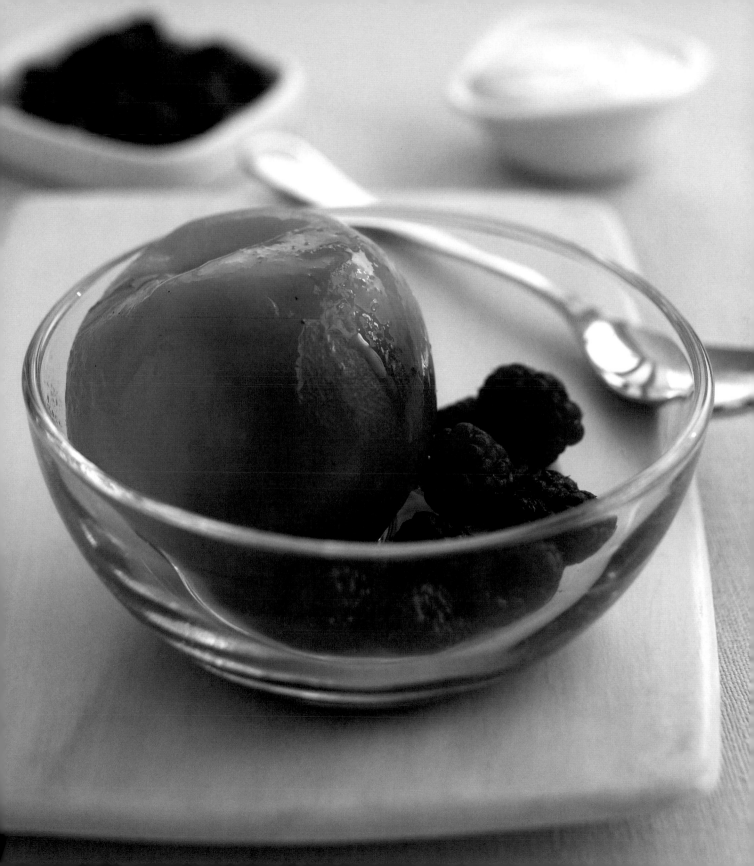

buckwheat blinis with ricotta and blueberries

Makes about 40 Preparation time: 10 minutes Cooking time: 10 minutes

1 cup buckwheat flour

¼ cup whole wheat flour

1½ teaspoons baking powder

2 tablespoons raw (demerara) sugar

2 eggs, lightly beaten

1 cup buttermilk

1 teaspoon vanilla extract

olive oil spray

low fat ricotta, to serve

fresh blueberries, to serve

These cute, bite-sized blinis would be great for a party. Alternatively, you could make them larger for a more substantial dessert.

1. Combine the flours, baking powder and sugar in a mixing bowl. Make a well in the center and pour in the eggs, buttermilk and vanilla, and whisk until smooth.
Add a little more milk if the batter is too thick.
2. Heat a frying pan over medium heat and lightly spray with oil. Drop the batter by the teaspoonful in batches, into the pan and cook for 1–2 minutes each side, or until the blinis are golden.
3. Serve topped with a teaspoon of ricotta and a few blueberries.

33 Cal, 1 g fat (saturated 1 g),
0 g fiber, 1 g protein, 5 g carbohydrate

bread and butter puddings

Serves 4 Preparation time: 10 minutes Cooking time: 30 minutes Standing time: 20 minutes

20 fl oz skim milk

4 eggs

½ cup Superfine sugar

2 teaspoons vanilla extract

3 slices sourdough bread,
  crusts removed

2 teaspoons polyunsaturated
  margarine

1 oz dried pear, finely chopped

¾ oz dried apricot,
  finely chopped

1 tablespoon apricot jam, warmed

powdered sugar, to dust

Fruit bread, instead of the sourdough, will also work well in these puddings.

1. Lightly butter four 1 cup ovenproof dishes.
2. Whisk the milk, eggs, sugar and vanilla together in a large mixing bowl.
3. Lightly spread one side of each sourdough slice with the margarine. Cut each slice into 4 triangles. Place 3 triangles into the base of each prepared dish, slightly overlapping to fit. Sprinkle over the dried fruit and pour over the milk mixture. Set aside for 15 minutes.
4. Preheat oven to 315°F.
5. Place the pudding dishes in a large, deep baking pan. Pour enough boiling water into the tray to come halfway up the sides of the dishes. Cover tray loosely with foil and bake for 15 minutes. Remove foil and continue to bake for 10 minutes. Remove pan from oven, brush the tops of the puddings with apricot jam and return to oven for another 5 minutes, or until puddings are golden and puffed.
6. Remove from oven and allow to cool for 5 minutes. Dust with powdered sugar and serve warm.

354 Cal, 7 g fat (saturated 2 g),
2 g fiber, 14 g protein, 59 g carbohydrate

baked raisin, date and walnut apples

Serves 4   Preparation time: 15 minutes   Macerating time: 2–3 hours   Cooking time: 30–40 minutes

⅓ cup raisins

⅓ cup dates, finely chopped

2 tablespoons port

olive oil spray

¼ cup walnuts, finely chopped

1 teaspoon finely grated orange zest

½ teaspoon ground cinnamon

pinch ground cloves

2 tablespoons brown sugar

4 large green apples, cored

1 cup apple juice

Baked apples make a fantastic winter dessert. Try serving them with low fat vanilla ice cream or yogurt. You can replace the port with orange juice, if you prefer.

1. Place raisins and dates in a small bowl, pour over the port and set aside to macerate for 2–3 hours.

2. Preheat oven to 350°F. Spray the bottom of a non-stick baking pan with a little oil.

3. Place the soaked fruit, walnuts, orange zest, spices and sugar in a medium-sized bowl and mix well.

4. Using a sharp knife, make a shallow cut horizontally around the middle of each apple (to prevent them from bursting during cooking). Stuff each with the fruit filling and place in the prepared pan. Pour the apple juice into the base of the pan.

5. Cover the baking tray loosely with foil and bake, basting the apples occasionally with the apple juice, for 30–40 minutes, or until apples are soft. Serve warm, with low fat vanilla ice cream or yogurt, if desired.

273 Cal, 6 g fat (saturated 0 g),
6 g fiber, 2 g protein, 50 g carbohydrate

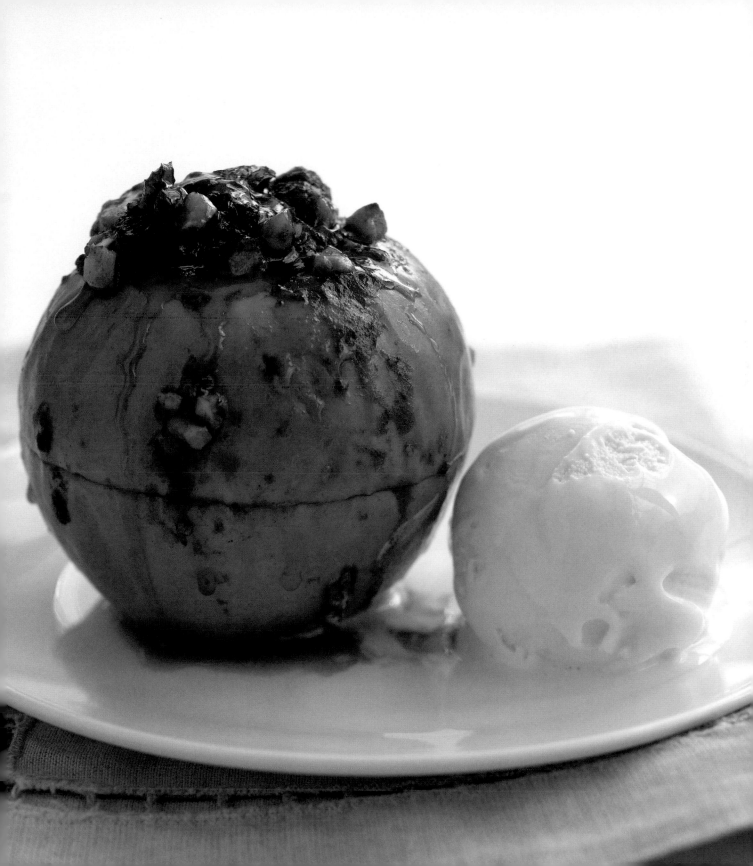

amaretti-baked nectarines

Serves 4   Preparation time: 10 minutes   Cooking time: 20 minutes

4 ripe nectarines
1¾ oz amaretti cookies
¼ cup almond meal
2 teaspoons brown sugar
1 egg yolk
1 tablespoon Marsala (optional)
1 tablespoon reduced fat margarine
powdered sugar, to dust
low fat vanilla yogurt, to serve

Baked nectarines are so delicious, yet so simple and quick to prepare. Any seasonal stone fruit, such as peaches or apricots, can be used in place of the nectarines. Amaretti are small macaroon-type cookies made from sweet and bitter almonds.

1. Preheat oven to 350°F.
2. Cut each nectarine in half and remove the stone. Place the amaretti cookies in a food processor and process until they resemble rough crumbs. Place in a medium-sized bowl with the almond meal, sugar, egg yolk and Marsala, if using, and mix until well combined.
3. Fill each nectarine with 2 teaspoons of the amaretti filling. Place the nectarines in a shallow, ovenproof dish and dot the top of each with a little margarine. Bake for 20 minutes, or until golden. Serve dusted with powdered sugar and a dollop of yogurt.

232 Cal, 10 g fat (saturated 3 g),
5 g fiber, 6 g protein, 27 g carbohydrate

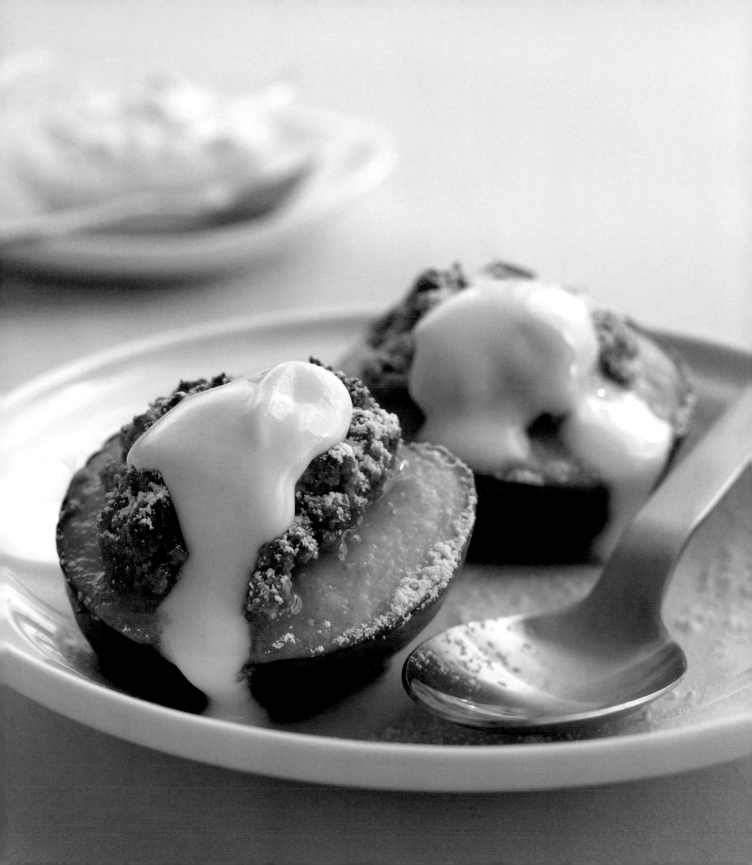

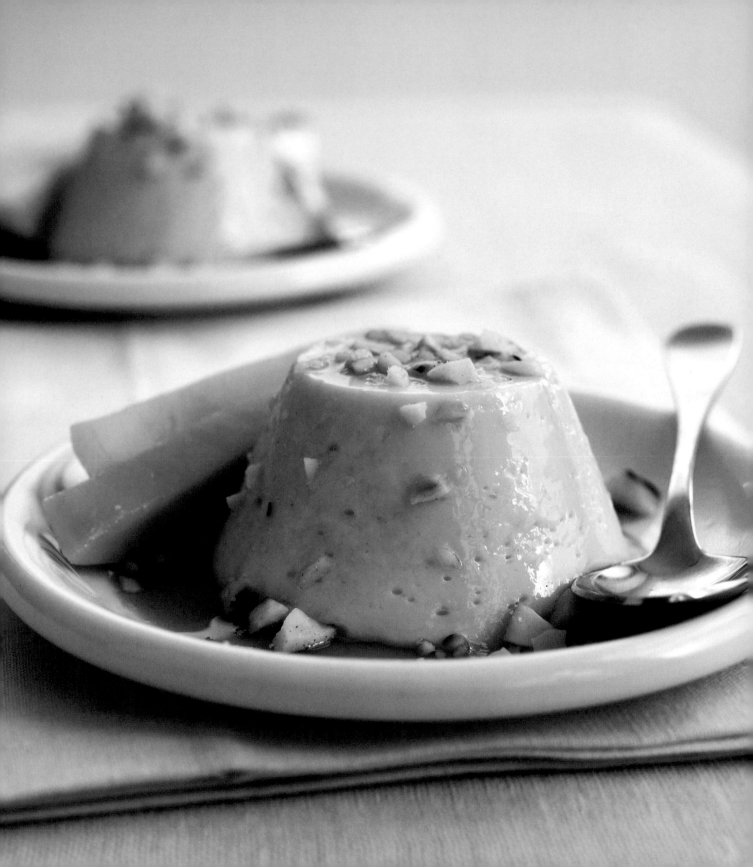

mango bavarois

Makes 4   Preparation: 20 minutes   Chilling time: overnight

7 oz fresh mango flesh

5½ oz silken tofu, chopped

1 cup buttermilk

2 tablespoons Superfine sugar

1 teaspoon vanilla extract

3 teaspoons gelatin

mango slices, extra, to serve

¼ cup macadamias, lightly roasted,
  chopped, to serve

maple syrup, to serve

This bavarois is delicious served with fresh fruit such as raspberries, blueberries or passionfruit.

1. Place the mango, tofu, buttermilk, sugar and vanilla in a blender, and blend on high until well combined. Leave mixture in blender.

2. Place 1 tablespoon water in a small bowl and sprinkle over the gelatin. Place the bowl into a larger bowl of boiling water (the boiling water should come halfway up the sides of the gelatin bowl). Stir the gelatin until dissolved. Set aside to cool.

3. Add the cooled gelatin mixture to the blender and blend on high for 1 minute. Place 4 x 5 fl oz dariole molds in a small baking dish. Divide the mixture evenly among the molds, cover with plastic wrap and refrigerate overnight.

4. When ready to serve, dip the base of each mold in hot water for 2 seconds, then carefully run a spatula around the edge of the mold. Invert the bavarois onto a serving plate, add the extra mango slices, sprinkle over the macadamias, and drizzle with a little maple syrup.

251 Cal, 13 g fat (saturated 2 g),
2 g fiber, 11 g protein, 24 g carbohydrate

creamy quinoa pudding

Serves 4–6 Preparation time: 10 minutes Cooking time: 40 minutes

¾ cup quinoa

2 cups low fat soy milk

1½ tablespoons Superfine sugar

1 cardamom pod, lightly crushed

juice and finely grated zest of 1 small
    orange

1 teaspoon vanilla extract

1 cinnamon stick

2 tablespoons honey

1 pomegranate, seeds scraped out

1. Rinse quinoa and place in a medium-sized saucepan with 2 cups water. Bring to a boil over high heat. Cover pan with a lid, lower heat and simmer for 15 minutes, or until the quinoa is tender and all the water is absorbed.

2. Add the soy milk, sugar, cardamom, orange zest, vanilla and cinnamon to the quinoa. Return to the boil, then reduce heat to low and cook, stirring frequently, for 15–20 minutes, or until the quinoa is creamy and the liquid is almost completely absorbed. Set aside.

3. Place the orange juice, honey and pomegranate seeds in a small saucepan and simmer for 3–4 minutes, or until slightly reduced.

4. Serve the warm quinoa pudding drizzled with a little of the pomegranate syrup.

COOK'S TIP

You could substitute quinoa with basmati rice in this recipe. There is no need to pre-cook the rice—just start at step 2 and allow a little more cooking time.

242 Cal, 3 g fat (saturated 0 g),
4 g fiber, 9 g protein, 47 g carbohydrate

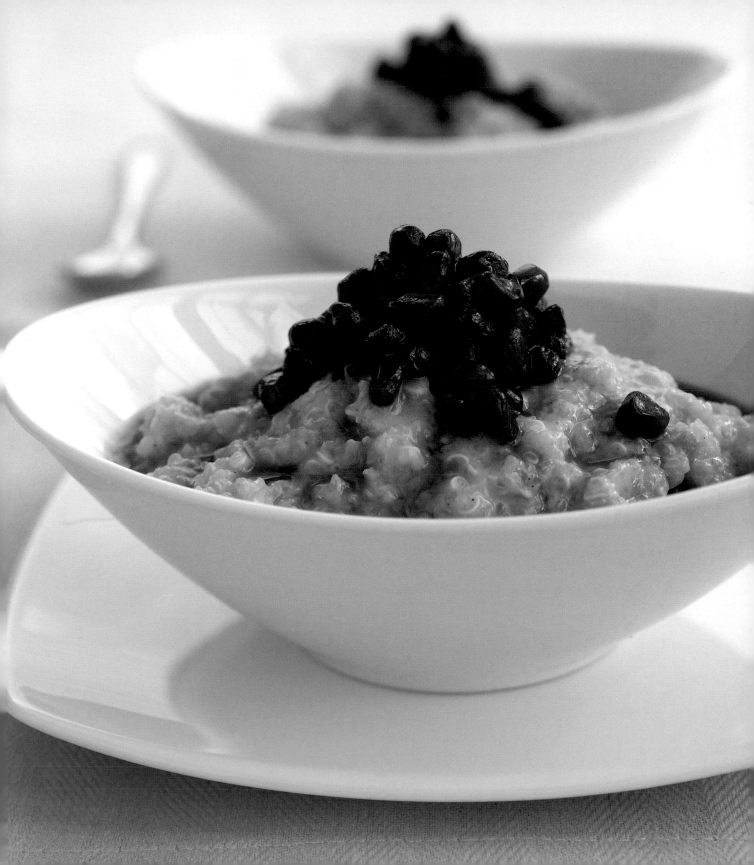

apple, rhubarb and ginger crumble

Serves 4 Preparation time: 10 minutes   Cooking time: 35 minutes   Cooling time: 5 minutes

14 oz (about 3 small) Granny Smith
 apples, peeled, cored, cut into thin
 wedges
1 small bunch (about 12 oz) rhubarb,
 ends trimmed, washed, cut into
 1½ in lengths
1 teaspoon finely grated ginger
2 tablespoons Superfine sugar
1 cinnamon stick

CRUMBLE
2 tablespoons plain flour
⅓ cup almond meal
3 tablespoons reduced fat margarine
½ cup rolled oats
¼ cup almonds, roughly chopped
3 tablespoons brown sugar
½ teaspoon ground ginger

1. Preheat oven to 350°F. Lightly grease a 6 cup ovenproof dish.

2. Place the apples, rhubarb, ginger, sugar and cinnamon with ⅔ cup water in a medium-sized saucepan. Simmer for 15 minutes, or until the apples and rhubarb are just cooked.

3. Meanwhile, for the crumble, place the flour and almond meal in a bowl. Use your fingertips to rub in the margarine until well combined and large crumbs form. Mix in the oats, almonds, sugar and ginger.

4. Spoon the fruit into the prepared dish and sprinkle the crumble over evenly. Bake for 20 minutes, or until golden and bubbling. Set aside to cool for 5 minutes before serving.

COOK'S TIP

This crumble can also be made as 4 individual crumbles. If rhubarb is unavailable, substitute extra apple.

368 Cal, 18 g fat (saturated 2 g),
7 g fiber, 7 g protein, 42 g carbohydrate

tofu and ricotta raspberry-swirl cheesecakes

Makes 6   Preparation time: 20 minutes   Cooking time: 1 hour 10 minutes   Chilling time: 3–4 hours

5 oz oatmeal cookies

3½ oz reduced fat margarine, melted

1 lb 2 oz reduced fat ricotta

9 oz silken tofu, well drained

finely grated rind of 1 lemon

1 teaspoon vanilla extract

3 eggs

½ cup pure floral honey or maple
  syrup

2 tablespoons good-quality
  raspberry jam

fresh raspberries, to serve

1. Preheat oven to 275°F. Line a 6 x 1 cup muffin tin with paper cups.

2. Place the cookies in a food processor and process until they form fine crumbs. Transfer to a bowl and stir in the margarine until well combined. Divide the mixture evenly among the paper cups and press down firmly to form a base. Place in the refrigerator while you make the filling.

3. Place the ricotta, tofu, lemon rind and vanilla in a food processor and process until smooth. Add the eggs and honey and beat until smooth and well combined.

4. Divide the ricotta mixture evenly among the prepared bases. Gently stir 1 teaspoon of jam into each cheesecake. Bake for 1 hour 10 minutes, or until just set in the middle.

5. Remove from oven and allow to cool completely before covering with plastic wrap and chilling for 3–4 hours. Serve topped with fresh raspberries.

474 Cal, 24 g fat (saturated 10 g),
2 g fiber, 18 g protein, 48 g carbohydrate

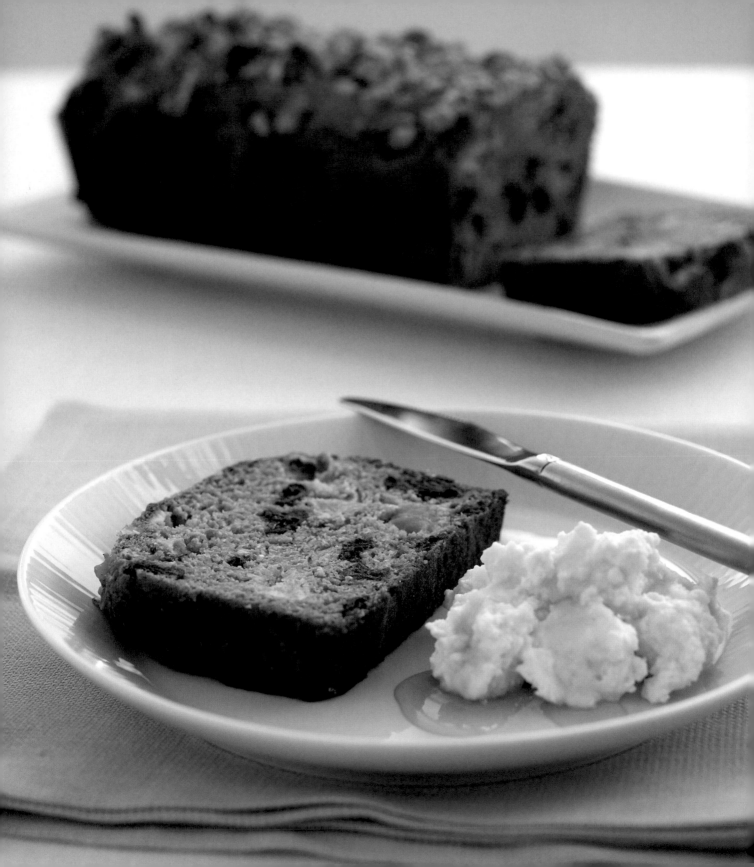

apple, cranberry and walnut bread

Makes 12 slices Preparation time: 10 minutes Soaking time: 30 minutes Cooking time: 45 minutes–1 hour

½ cup rolled oats

10 fl oz skim milk

1½ cups self-rising whole wheat flour

1 teaspoon baking powder

4½ oz dried cranberries

⅔ cup firmly packed dried apple, cut
  into small dice

⅓ cup brown sugar

1 teaspoon ground cinnamon

½ teaspoon allspice

⅓ cup pure floral honey

¼ cup walnuts, finely chopped

This loaf makes a fantastic breakfast when toasted and topped with a little low fat ricotta and honey.

1. Place the rolled oats in a bowl, pour over the milk and set aside to soak for 30 minutes.
2. Preheat oven to 350°F.
3. Sift the flour and baking powder into a large bowl. Add the oat mixture, cranberries, apple, sugar, spices and honey and mix well to combine.
4. Spoon the mixture into a 2 lb non-stick (or greased) loaf tin, smoothing the top with a spatula. Sprinkle with the walnuts. Bake for 45 minutes–1 hour or until golden brown and a skewer inserted into the centre comes out clean.
5. Remove from oven and allow to cool a little in the tin before turning out onto a wire rack to cool completely. The loaf will store for several weeks if wrapped in foil and kept in an airtight container.

COOK'S TIP

Substitute any of your favorite dried fruits for the dried apple and cranberries.

211 Cal, 3 g fat (saturated 0 g),
4 g fiber, 5 g protein, 41 g carbohydrate

carob, ginger and pecan biscotti

Makes about 50 Preparation time: 10 minutes Cooking time: 40 minutes

⅔ cup Superfine sugar

2 eggs

1¼ cup all-purpose whole wheat flour

½ cup carob powder

2 tablespoons glacé ginger, finely
  chopped

⅓ cup pecans

⅓ cup almonds

These delicious little cookies are perfect for serving with coffee.

1. Preheat oven to 350°F. Line a large baking tray with baking paper.
2. Using electric beaters, beat the sugar and eggs together for 3 minutes, or until thick, pale and increased in volume. Sift in the flour and carob powder and stir with a wooden spoon until almost combined. Add the ginger and nuts, and use a clean hand to mix until well combined.
3. Divide the mixture in half and shape into 2 logs about 6 in long. Place on the prepared tray and flatten slightly to ¾ in thick. Bake for 20 minutes, or until firm. Remove from the oven and allow to cool completely.
4. Preheat oven to 250°F. Cut the logs into slices about ⅓ in thick. Spread out in a single layer onto oven trays and bake, turning once, for 20 minutes. Transfer biscotti to wire racks to cool completely before serving. They can be stored in an airtight container for up to 1 month.

COOK'S TIP

You can substitute cocoa for the carob powder, if desired.

42 Cal, 1 g fat (saturated 0 g),
1 g fiber, 1 g protein, 6 g carbohydrate

chewy fig and apricot granola bars

Makes 12 Preparation time: 10 minutes Cooking time: 15–20 minutes

½ cup self-rising flour

½ cup all-purpose whole wheat flour

⅓ cup almond meal

1 teaspoon baking powder

½ teaspoon mixed spice

½ teaspoon ground cinnamon

1¼ cups rolled oats

½ cup dried apricots, chopped

½ cup dried figs, chopped

¼ cup sunflower seeds

½ cup apple juice

¼ cup vegetable oil

1 egg, lightly beaten

2 egg whites, lightly beaten

2 tablespoons pure floral honey

Children (and adults) will love these granola bars.

1. Preheat oven to 375°F. Line an 8 x 12 in slice pan with baking paper.

2. Sift the flours, almond meal, baking powder and spices into a large bowl. Stir in the oats, dried fruit and sunflower seeds. Add the apple juice, oil and whole egg, and mix well. Gently mix in the egg whites until just combined.

3. Press the mixture evenly and firmly into the prepared pan with the back of a spoon. Using a sharp knife, mark the 12 bars into the surface.

4. Bake for 15–20 minutes, or until golden brown. Remove from oven and allow to cool before cutting into bars.

COOK'S TIP

The dried apricot and fig could be replaced with other dried fruits, such as pear, dates and apple. These bars are suitable to freeze.

219 Cal, 9 g fat (saturated 1 g),
4 g fiber, 5 g protein, 27 g carbohydrate

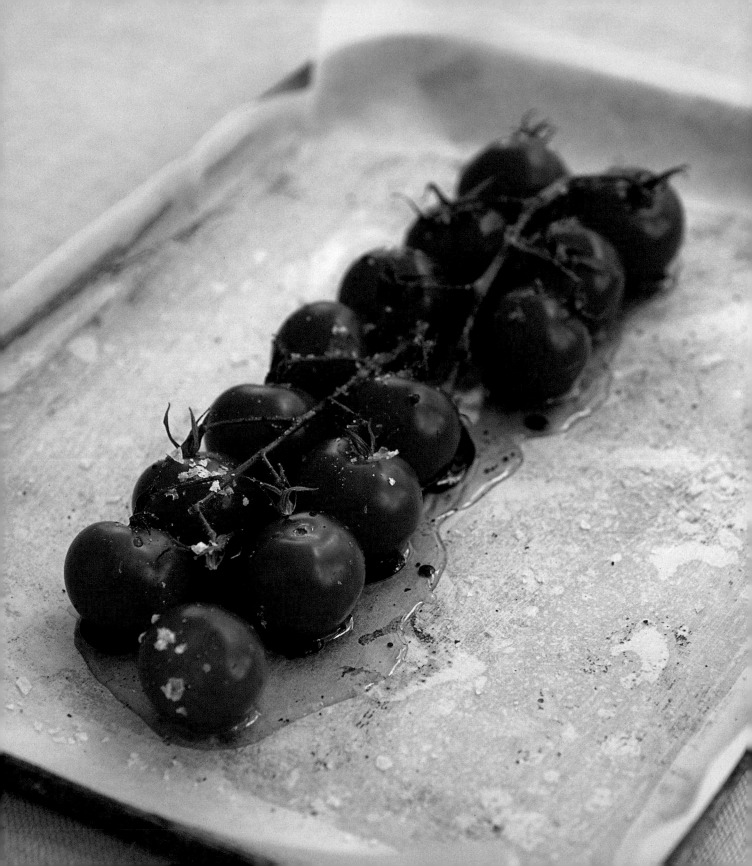

basics

Salsas, sauces, salads and spice mixes—use your pantry essentials to create quick and satisfying snacks or to add the final flourish to a recipe. You'll soon incorporate these indispensable, fail-safe basics into your everyday routine.

YOGURT TAHINI DRESSING

½ cup low fat natural yogurt

1 teaspoon tahini

2 teaspoons lemon juice

1 teaspoon pure floral honey or pinch caster sugar

1. Whisk all ingredients together until well combined.

One tablespoon serving:
12 Cal, 1 g fat (saturated 0 g),
1 g fiber, 1 g protein, 2 g carbohydrate

HERBIE'S TAGINE SPICE MIX

5 teaspoons mild paprika

2½ teaspoons ground cilantro

1 teaspoon ground cinnamon

1 teaspoon medium-heat chili powder

½ teaspoon ground allspice

¼ teaspoon ground cloves

¼ teaspoon ground green cardamom seeds

1. Blend all spices and store in an airtight container.

Recipe: Ian Hemphill, www.herbies.com.au

CASABLANCAN COUSCOUS

Serves 4 Preparation time: 10 minutes

Cooking time: 20 minutes   Standing time: 10 minutes

2 cups couscous

½ teaspoon salt

2 teaspoons sunflower oil

2 teaspoons reduced fat margarine

1 tablespoon finely chopped preserved lemon

1. Preheat oven to 400°F.

2. Place the couscous in a bowl. Stir the salt into 400 ml (13 fl oz) warm water, then pour it over the couscous, stirring to make sure it is absorbed evenly. Leave to stand for 10 minutes. Using your fingertips, rub the sunflower oil into the grains to air them and break up any clumps. Tip the couscous into an ovenproof dish, dot with the margarine, cover with foil and place in the oven for about 20 minutes.

3. Remove the couscous from the oven. Use a fork to fluff it up, mix in the preserved lemon, then pile onto a serving dish.

378 Cal, 5 g fat (saturated 1 g),
1 g fiber, 12 g protein, 70 g carbohydrate

CHILE CORN SALSA

Serves 4 Preparation time: 10 minutes

Cooking time: 12 minutes

2 corn cobs

2 vine-ripened tomatoes, seeded, cut into small dice

½ red onion, finely chopped

1 small red pepper, deseeded, finely chopped

2 small red chiles, deseeded, finely chopped

2 tablespoons finely chopped chives

2 tablespoons finely chopped cilantro

1 tablespoon red-wine vinegar

1 tablespoon lime juice

1 tablespoon olive oil

pinch Superfine sugar

salt and freshly ground black pepper

1. Steam or boil the corn cobs until tender, then drain.

2. Using a sharp knife, cut the kernels from the cobs and place in a large bowl. Add the tomato, onion, pepper, chile, chives and cilantro.

3. In a separate bowl, whisk together the vinegar, lime juice, oil and sugar. Toss the dressing through the salsa, and season.

140 Cal, 6 g fat (saturated 1 g),
4 g fiber, 4 g protein, 16 g carbohydrate

TOMATO AND BEAN SALSA

Serves 4 Preparation time: 5 minutes

Cooking time: 1 hour

1 tablespoon olive oil

1 small onion, finely chopped

1 small red chile, deseeded, finely chopped

3 cloves garlic, crushed

1 teaspoon ground cumin

½ teaspoon sweet paprika

2 – 14 oz cans chopped tomatoes

1 – 14 oz can red kidney beans, rinsed and drained

3 tablespoons chopped flat-leaf parsley

1. Heat the oil in a medium-sized saucepan over medium heat. Add the onion and chile and cook, stirring, for 5 minutes, or until onion is soft. Add the garlic, cumin and paprika and cook, stirring, for a further 2 minutes.

2. Add the tomatoes, bring to the boil, then reduce the heat and simmer for 30 minutes. Add the kidney beans, return to the boil, then reduce the heat and simmer for a further 20 minutes. Stir in the parsley. Set aside to cool before serving. The salsa will keep in an airtight container in the fridge for 2–3 days.

158 Cal, 5 g fat (saturated 1 g),
7 g fiber, 6 g protein, 17 g carbohydrate

HUMMUS

Serves 6 (makes 1½ cups)

1⅓ cups cooked chickpeas
¼ cup tahini
2 cloves garlic
3 tablespoons fresh lemon juice
2 tablespoons olive oil
salt and freshly ground black pepper

Place all ingredients except salt and pepper in a small food processor. Process until well combined and smooth. Add 2–3 tablespoons hot water to thin the mixture slightly, and season. The hummus will keep in an airtight container in the fridge for up to 2 weeks.

108 Cal, 14 g fat (saturated 1 g),
2 g fiber, 3 g protein, 6 g carbohydrate

TABBOULEH

Serves 6 (makes 3 cups)

¾ cup bulgur wheat
1 cup firmly packed, picked flat-leaf parsley leaves, finely chopped
1 cup firmly packed, picked mint leaves, finely shredded
1 small red (Spanish) onion, finely chopped
2 ripe tomatoes, finely chopped
¼ cup fresh lemon juice
2 tablespoons olive oil
salt and freshly ground black pepper

1. Place the bulgur in a small heatproof bowl and cover with 6½ fl oz hot water. Set aside for 20 minutes.
2. Place the bulgur in a bowl with the parsley, mint, onion and tomato, and toss to combine. In a separate small bowl, whisk together the lemon juice and oil, and season. Add to the tabbouleh and toss to combine. The tabbouleh will keep in an airtight container in the fridge for 2–3 days.

147 Cal, 7 g fat (saturated fat 1 g),
5 g fiber, 4 g protein, 16 g carbohydrate

SPICY TOMATO SAUCE

Serves 4 (makes 1¼ cups)

2 teaspoons olive oil
1 onion, finely chopped
1 clove garlic, crushed
1 small, fresh red chile, finely chopped
1 – 14 oz can chopped tomatoes
½ cup good-quality vegetable stock
pinch sugar
salt and freshly ground black pepper

Heat the oil in a small saucepan over medium heat. Add the onion, garlic and chile and cook, stirring, for 5–6 minutes, or until softened. Add the tomatoes and stock and bring to a simmer. Simmer, uncovered, for 15–20 minutes, or until the sauce reduces and thickens. Add sugar, and season. The sauce will keep in an airtight container in the fridge for up to 1 week.

47 Cal, 3 g fat (saturated 1 g),
1 g fiber, 1 g protein, 4 g carbohydrate

BARLEY AND RED RICE SALAD

Serves 4 Preparation time: 10 minutes
Cooking time: 45 minutes

½ cup pearl barley
1 teaspoon dried dill
3½ oz red rice
2 teaspoons olive oil
4 scallions, trimmed, finely sliced
1 in piece fresh ginger, peeled,
  finely grated
1 clove garlic, crushed

You can substitute the red rice with wild rice or brown rice, if you prefer.

1. Cook the pearl barley in a large saucepan of boiling water. Add the dill and simmer for 30–35 minutes, or until tender. Drain well. Meanwhile, cook the rice in a separate saucepan of boiling water for 35 minutes, or until tender. Drain well.
2. Heat the oil in a large non-stick frying pan over medium heat. Add the scallions, ginger and garlic and cook, stirring, for 1–2 minutes, or until fragrant. Add the pearl barley and rice and cook, stirring, for a further 12 minutes, or until heated through.

197 Cal, 4 g fat (saturated 1 g),
4 g fiber, 4 g protein, 35 g carbohydrate

your low GI diet foods

To make easy low GI choices, you'll need to stock the right foods. Here are ideas for what to keep in your pantry, refrigerator and freezer. These foods have optimum flavor and nutritional value and can all feature in a low GI healthy eating plan.

What to keep in your pantry

Asian sauces Hoi sin, soy and tamari are a good basic range.

Barley One of the oldest cultivated cereals, barley is very nutritious and high in soluble fiber. Look for products such as pearl barley to use in soups, stews and pilafs or rolled barley as an alternative to traditional oatmeal.

Black pepper Buy freshly ground pepper, or grind your own peppercorns.

Bread Low GI options include grainy, stone-ground wholemeal, pumpernickel, sourdough, whole grain English-style muffins, flat bread and pita bread.

Breakfast cereals These include traditional rolled oats, natural muesli and low GI packaged breakfast cereals.

Bulgur wheat Use it to make tabbouleh, or add to veggie burgers, stuffings, soups and stews.

Canned evaporated skim milk This makes an excellent substitute for cream in pasta sauces.

Canned fruit Have a variety of canned fruit on hand, including peaches, pears, apples and nectarines—choose the brands labelled with "no added sugar".

Canned vegetables Sweet corn kernels and tomatoes can help to boost the vegetable content of a meal. Tomatoes, in particular, can be used freely because they are rich in antioxidants, as well as having a low GI. Choose low salt or "no added salt" varieties.

Couscous Ready in minutes; serve with casseroles and braised dishes.

Curry pastes A tablespoon or so makes a delicious curry base.

Dried fruit These include raisins, apricots, prunes and apples.

Dried herbs Oregano, basil, ground coriander, thyme and rosemary can be useful to have on stand-by in the pantry.

Honey Try to avoid the commercial honeys or honey blends, and use the pure floral honeys instead. These varieties have a much lower GI. Bioactive components in these honeys appear to reduce their GI naturally.

Jam A dollop of good-quality jam (with no added sugar) on toast contains fewer calories than butter or margarine.

Legumes Stock a variety of legumes (dried or canned), including lentils, split peas and beans. There are many bean varieties, including cannellini, butter, cranberry, kidney and soy beans.

Maple syrup A sweetener made from the sap

of maple trees which can be used in place of honey in a vegan diet. Used in baking and desserts, pure maple syrup has a low GI. (Imitation varieties have a higher GI.)

Mustard Seeded or whole grain mustard is useful as a sandwich spread, and in salad dressings and sauces.

Noodles Many Asian noodles, such as hokkien, udon and rice vermicelli, have low to medium GI values because of their dense texture, whether they are made from wheat or rice flour.

Nuts Eat a handful of nuts (about 30 g/1 oz) every other day. Try them sprinkled over your breakfast cereal, salad or dessert, and enjoy unsalted nuts as a snack as well.

Oils Use olive oil for general use; extra-virgin for salad dressings, marinades and dishes that benefit from its flavor; and sesame oil for Asian-style stir-fries. Canola or olive oil cooking sprays are handy too.

Pasta A great source of carbohydrates and B vitamins. Fresh or dried, the preparation is easy. Simply cook in boiling water until just tender, or al dente, drain and top with your favorite sauce and a sprinkle of vegetarian cheese.

Quinoa This whole grain cooks in about 10–15 minutes and has a slightly chewy texture. It can be used as a substitute for rice, couscous or bulgur wheat. It is very important to rinse the grains thoroughly before cooking.

Rice Basmati or Japanese koshihikari varieties are good choices because they have a lower GI than, for example, jasmine or white rice.

Rolled oats Beside their use in oatmeal, oats can be added to cakes, biscuits, breads and desserts.

Sea salt Use in moderation. Iodized sea salt is a preferred source of iodine for vegetarians.

Seeds Pumpkin seeds, sunflower seeds, sesame seeds and flaxseeds are full of the good fats and make useful sprinkles to add to stir-fries, salads or muesli. Try roasting them tossed in a little tamari sauce.

Spices Most spices, including ground cumin, turmeric, cinnamon, paprika and nutmeg, should be bought in small quantities because they lose pungency with age and incorrect storage.

Stock Make your own stock or buy ready-made vegetable stock, which is available in long-life cartons in the supermarket. To keep the sodium content down with ready-made stocks, look out for a low salt option.

Tofu, tempeh and TVP Keep these useful protein foods on hand to add to stir-fries, salads and casseroles. Either marinate them yourself or buy ready-marinated varieties.

Tomato paste Use in soups, sauces and casseroles. Choose "no added salt" varieties.

Vinegar White-wine or red-wine vinegar and balsamic vinegar are excellent as vinaigrette dressings in salads.

What to keep in your refrigerator

Bottled vegetables Sun-dried tomatoes, olives, grilled eggplant and pepper are handy to keep as flavorsome additions to pastas and sandwiches.

Capers and olives These can be bought in jars and kept in the refrigerator once opened. They are a tasty (but salty) addition to pizzas, salads and pasta dishes.

Cheese Any reduced fat vegetarian cheese is great to keep handy in the refrigerator. A block of parmesan is indispensable and will keep for up to 1 month. Reduced fat cottage and ricotta cheeses have a short life so are best bought as needed, and can be a good alternative to butter or margarine in a sandwich.

Condiments Keep jars of minced garlic, chili or ginger in the refrigerator to spice up your cooking in an instant.

Eggs To enhance your intake of omega–3 fats, we suggest using omega–3-enriched eggs. Although the yolk is high in cholesterol, the fat in eggs is predominantly monounsaturated, and therefore considered a "good" fat.

Fresh herbs These are available in most supermarkets and there really is no substitute for the flavor they impart. For variety, try parsley, basil, mint, chives and coriander.

Fresh fruit Almost all fruits make an excellent low GI snack. When in season, try fruit such as apples, oranges, pears, grapes, grapefruit, peaches, apricots, strawberries and mangoes.

Milk Skim or low fat milk is best, or try low fat calcium-enriched soy milk.

Vegetables Keep a variety of seasonal vegetables on hand, such as spinach, broccoli cauliflower, Asian greens, asparagus, zucchini and mushrooms. Pepper, spring onions and sprouts (mung bean and snow pea sprouts) are great to bulk up a salad. Corn, sweet potato and yam are essential to your low GI food store.

Yogurt Low fat natural yogurt provides the most calcium for the fewest calories. Have vanilla or fruit versions as a dessert, or use natural yogurt as a condiment in savoury dishes. However, if using yogurt in a hot meal, make sure you add it at the last minute, and do not let it boil, otherwise it will curdle.

What to keep in your freezer

Frozen berries Berries can make any dessert special, and by using frozen ones it means you don't have to wait until berry season in order to indulge. Try berries such as blueberries, raspberries and strawberries.

Frozen vegetables Keep a packet of peas, beans, corn, spinach or mixed vegetables in the freezer—these are handy to add to a quick meal.

Frozen yogurt This is a fantastic substitute for ice cream, and some products even have a similar creamy texture, but with much less fat.

Ice cream Reduced or low fat ice cream is ideal for a quick dessert, served with fresh fruit.

Making sense of food labelling

These days, food labels contain a lot of detailed information, but unfortunately few people know how to interpret it correctly. Often the claims on the package don't mean quite what you think. Here are some prime examples:

- **Cholesterol free** Take care, as the food may still be high in fat.
- **Reduced fat** Double-check if the product is actually low in fat. Even though the fat content may be reduced, it may still be very high.
- **No added sugar** This does not necessarily mean that a product is low in sugar—it could still raise your blood glucose levels.
- **Lite or light** Check to see exactly what the product is light in. The "lite" could simply mean light in color.

How do you know if a product is low, medium or high GI?

Low GI eating often means making a move back to staple foods—fruit, vegetables, legumes, whole grains, pasta, noodles, dairy foods—which naturally have a low GI, so it doesn't matter which brand you buy. When it comes to carbohydrate-rich processed foods such as breakfast cereals, bread and bakery items, the GI can range from low to high depending on the brand. To find the GI of your favourite brands you can:

- Look for an independently accredited GI symbol on the product.
- Check the nutritional label. Some manufacturers now include GI (but you need to be sure that an accredited lab tested the food).
- Visit www.glycemicindex.com to search the database.
- Contact the manufacturer and ask them to have the food tested by an accredited lab.

The GI Symbol Program

This international symbol is a guarantee that the product meets strict nutritional criteria. Glycemic Index Limited is a non-profit company established to run the GI Symbol Program. Its members are: the University of Sydney, Diabetes Australia and the Juvenile Diabetes Research Foundation. For more information, visit www.gisymbol.com.

Acknowledgments

We would like to thank Ian Hofstetter and Katy Holder for their beautiful food photography; Chrissy Freer and Alison Roberts for taking our food ideas, testing them and creating delicious recipes and Ellie Exarchos for designing this lovely book and for her willingness to take on board our thoughts about how it should look! But, most of all we would like to thank the two special people who really pulled it all together and made it happen—our publisher, Fiona Hazard, and production editor, Anna Waddington, at Hachette Livre Australia.

About the authors

JENNIE BRAND-MILLER, PHD, one of the world's leading authorities on carbohydrates and the glycemic index, has championed the GI approach to nutrition for more than 20 years. Professor of Nutrition at the University of Sydney and a former President of the Nutrition Society of Australia, she is an in-demand speaker on the GI and her laboratory at the University of Sydney is the world's foremost GI-testing center.

KAYE FOSTER-POWELL, M NUTR & DIET, RD, is an accredited practicing dietitian with extensive experience in diabetes management, is the co-author, with Dr. Brand-Miller, of the authoritative tables of GI and glycemic load values published in the *American Journal of Clinical Nutrition*.

KATE MARSH, M NUTR & DIET, RD, is an accredited practicing dietitian and diabetes educator in Sydney, with particular expertise in vegetarian nutrition. She chairs the Dietitian's Association of Australia Vegetarian Interest Group and writes for the Australian Vegetarian Society Magazine. Marsh is currently undertaking her PhD at the University of Sydney and is co-author of *The New Glucose Revolution Guide to Living Well with PCOS*.

PHILIPPA SANDALL is a writer and editor who specializes in the areas of food, health, and nutrition and has been involved in the Glucose Revolution series since its inception in 1996.

Websites for more information on GI:
The GI database: www.glycemicindex.com
The official glycemic index monthly newsletter: www.ginews.blogspot.com
The GI Symbol Program: www.gisymbol.com

Index

Although every effort has been made to ensure that the contents of this book are accurate, it must not be treated as a substitute for qualified medical advice. Always consult a qualified medical practitioner. Neither the authors nor the publisher can be held responsible for any loss or claim arising out of the use, or misuse, of the suggestions made or the failure to take medical advice.